MENTAL HEALTH AT THE CROSSROADS

Mental Health at the Crossroads
The Promise of the Psychosocial Approach

Edited by

SHULAMIT RAMON
Anglia Polytechnic University, Cambridge, UK

JANET E. WILLIAMS
Sheffield Hallam University, UK

ASHGATE

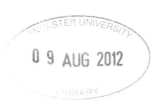
C1.
IMG
⟨M⟩

Published by
Ashgate Publishing Limited
Gower House
Croft Road
Aldershot
Hants GU11 3HR
England

Ashgate Publishing Company
Suite 420
101 Cherry Street
Burlington, VT 05401-4405
USA

Ashgate website: http://www.ashgate.com

British Library Cataloguing in Publication Data
Mental health at the crossroads : the promise of the
    psychosocial approach
    1. Mental health services - Social aspects 2. Mental illness
    3. Mental health policy
    I. Ramon, Shulamit II. Williams, Janet E.
    362.2'042

Library of Congress Cataloging-in-Publication Data
Mental health at the crossroads : the promise of the psychosocial approach / edited by Shulamit Ramon and Janet E. Williams.
        p. ; cm.
    Includes bibliographical references and index.
    ISBN 0-7546-4191-0 (alk. paper)
    1. Mental health services--Cross-cultural studies. 2. Mental health policy--Cross-cultural studies. 3. Social psychology--Methodology.
    [DNLM: 1. Mental Health Services--trends. 2. Cross-Cultural Comparison. 3. Health Policy--trends. 4. Psychology, Social--methods. WM 30 M54435 2005] I. Ramon, Shulamit. II. Williams, Janet E. 1951-

    RA790.M3623 2005
    362.2--dc22

                                                                    2005007433

ISBN 0 7546 4191 0

Printed and bound in Great Britain by MPG Books Ltd. Bodmin, Cornwall.

Contents

List of Contributors

Prof. Phil Barker is a former psychiatric nurse, Visiting Professor in Health Science at Trinity College Dublin and a psychotherapist in private practice who has researched and published on behavioural interventions, spirituality and user involvement in mental health.

Poppy Buchanan-Barker is a former social worker, and presently the Director of Clan Unity International, a mental health recovery agency based in Scotland.

Prof. Peter Beresford is a mental health service user activist, Professor of Social Policy and Director of the Centre for Citizen Participation of Brunel University, Chair of Shaping Our Lives, a Visiting Professor at the University of East Anglia, and a member of SCIE partnership council. He has published extensively on citizen and user participation.

Prof. Thomasina Borkman is Professor of Anthropology and Sociology at George Mason University, Washington DC, US. She has researched extensively and published on self-help and mutual support internationally, focusing on the history, concepts and theories of these issues.

Dr. Duncan Double is a consultant psychiatrist working for the NHS in Norwich, and a senior lecturer in the medical school at the East Anglia University. One of the founders of the Critical Psychiatry Network, he has researched the historical origins of the biopsychosocial approach, and has written in-depth about traditional psychiatry.

Neil Foster is currently a team manager working in a mental health partnership trust in the UK. He is a social worker and an ASW (approved under the 1983 Mental Health Act) and has managed ASW teams for seven years. He has visited community teams and in-patient facilities in the USA and in Australia and is currently engaged in comparative research in relation to forms of assertive outreach in all three counties.

Catherine Gamble is nurse consultant, St. George's Medical School, London. A nurse educationalist, she has developed and taught the Thorn course on psychosocial interventions in South Bank University and Oxfordshire mental health care trust, and published about psychosocial interventions with individuals and families.

Prof. Bill Healy is Associate Professor of Social Work at La Trobe University, Melbourne, Australia. A senior trainer and researcher at North Western Mental

Health Service in Melbourne, he researched and published on Australian and international issues of mental health social work and policy.

Dr. Julia Jones is a senior researcher in mental health at City University College, who has been until recently Marie Curie research fellow in Verona University, Italy, following a number of years at the Royal College of Nursing Research Unit in Oxford. Julia is a nurse and geographer, who researched issues such as the quality of care on acute wards, the educational needs of qualified mental health nurses, and collaborative research between users and professionals in mental health.

Dr. Roberto Mezzina is a consultant psychiatrist, and director of the Barcola Mental Health Centre in Trieste, Italy. Roberto has initiated user involvement in the centre, researched crisis issues and responses to them, and has published extensively on the Italian Psychiatric Reform.

Dr. Carol Munn-Giddings is reader in participatory action research at Anglia Polytechnic University, who has researched and published on this research modality. Carol has been researching self and mutual help with Tomasina Borkman internationally, including user-led initiatives.

Prof. David Pilgrim is Rathbone Professor of Sociology of Mental Health at Liverpool University. The Clinical Dean of the Teaching Primary Care Trust for East Lancashire, he has researched and published extensively on psychosocial issues and users' views of mental health services, especially the critique of traditional psychiatry from a sociological perspective.

Dr. Pauline Prior is senior lecturer in social policy at Queen's University, Belfast. She has researched and published on a wide range of issues in relation to mental health policy, such as gender, law and history in the UK and Europe.

Prof. Shulamit Ramon is Professor of Inter-Professional Health and Social Studies at Anglia Polytechnic University. A social worker and clinical psychologist by training, she has researched and published extensively on innovation in European mental health, psychosocial critique of the traditional psychiatry, mental health social work, user and carer involvement in training and research.

Dr. Joan Rapaport has a social work background and has worked in child care and mental health settings, and has researched in depth the place of carers in the British mental health system. She is currently working at the Social Workforce Research Unit at Kings College.

Dr. Noel Renouf is chief social worker, Northern Area Mental Health services, Melbourne, and senior lecturer at the school of social work at Latrobe University. With Ryan and Healy, he has researched internationally mental health social work and contributed to research on the role of the consumer consultant.

Dr. Eduardo Mourão Vasconcelos is senior lecturer in mental health policy at the School of Social Work and the Institute of Psychiatry in the University of Rio de Janiero, Brazil. A psychologist and political scientist by background, he has been a major leading figure of the Brazilian mental health reform. Eduardo has researched and published extensively on lay perceptions of mental illness, mental health policy and its reform, both in Brazil and in the UK.

Dr. Jan Wallcraft is a Fellow of the National Institute for Mental Health in England, responsible for ensuring a voice for Experts in Experience. She is also a senior researcher for user-focussed research at the Sainsbury Centre for Mental Health, who has researched the pathways to recovery from the perspective of service users.

Janet E. Williams is senior lecturer in social work at the Faculty of Health and Wellbeing, Sheffield Hallam University. Within mental health she worked in an innovative and participatory project in Chesterfield. She researches gender, service user involvement and service responses to women survivors of childhood sexual abuse, her publications are in social work education with a focus on learning in international contexts.

Foreword

The title of this book suggests that we are at a choice point. This is not for the first time. For the past hundred years a core contradiction has been replayed, creating recurrent versions of 'crossroads' and 'promise'. 'Crisis' also comes to mind – can a crisis be permanent? If one stays around long enough in mental health debates a sense of *déjà vu* becomes the norm. On the one hand, dominant interests arising from the interplay of professional power, industrial profit, governmental control and public prejudice have been evident. On the other hand this constellation of interests has encountered resistance, some of it reaching popular endorsement, albeit temporarily. The resistance reflects subordinate interests, especially in relation to the struggle for full citizenship for those with mental health problems.

Recently, in our British context, there has been a sense of a progressive push being obstructed by the strong authoritarian streak, which has characterised so much of the New Labour project. Its authoritarianism is surpassed only by its love affair with all things American – not only in relation to military adventurism, but also in our government's tendency to lift US social policies off the shelf for adoration and implementation. The recent attempt to reform mental health law, to shift powers of coercive control into the community, mirrors versions of a policy already implemented in many States in the USA.

Neil Foster's chapter on risk policies and citizenship in Australia, the UK and the US, and that of Bill Healy on Australian policies, amplify well the tension between these issues.

A measure of how bad it has become is that the Royal College of Psychiatrists has signed up to a multi-party alliance to oppose government intentions. In the run up to previous legislation, psychiatrists may not have got everything they wanted, at the time, but their tactics were of quiet negotiation, not public opposition. A switch to the latter suggests that either the legitimation crisis of the profession now demands more desperate measures or the government has misjudged the mood of many who have been involved in mental health debates for far longer than its ministers (or both).

Psychiatrists have developed a bad name with some good reason. But, as some in this book highlight, it is important to distinguish stereotypes from norms. The norm has been for the psychiatric profession to pursue a long term and defensive campaign to make itself respectable as a medical specialism. The first initiative was to assert (and keep asserting) that madness is a brain disease. The second was to shift its empire of beds from large Dickensian hospitals to shiny District General acute units. Twenty years on the shine has disappeared from these non-therapeutic holding centres for risky people. More recently psychiatry has embarked upon a clever strategy to de-stigmatise and thereby legitimise mental illness. The bio-medical paternalistic norm in the profession still privileges the doctor's right to treat over the patient's right to freedom.

Having said all of these critical things about the psychiatric profession, certain caveats in its defence are needed to challenge a stereotype. No other profession in the 'psy complex' has produced the volume (in both senses) of intellectual and political leadership required to challenge its own conservative norms and self-interest. Freud, Meyer, Sullivan, Menninger, Laing, Cooper, Szasz, Basaglia, Romme have all been shining lights. As Duncan Double's chapter shows, the work of Adolf Meyer in particular pre-dated the use by George Engel of general systems theory to codify the 'biopsychosocial' model.

Roberto Mezzina, practising psychiatry in Trieste, outlines in the book the evolving post-Basaglia radical social psychiatry.

Moreover, the users' movement has been aided in its efforts by this list of psychiatric radicals. Its resistance to the discourse of 'mental illness' can be traced to the work of Thomas Szasz. The right to find meaning in madness, asserted latterly by the Hearing Voices Network, resonates with the work of Ronald Laing and Marius Romme. These links suggest that stereotyping is unreasonable, when it is about psychiatrists not just their patients. In the other direction, it makes it difficult for the psychiatric orthodoxy to characterise 'anti-psychiatry' as some sort of external, hostile campaign, populated wholly by envious competing professionals or radical social scientists. The term was embraced by few to whom it was applied – maybe only David Cooper. It seems that people do not like being labelled but, more importantly, most of those called 'anti-psychiatrists' were *psychiatrists*. The 'enemy' maybe, but it has been within not without.

This tension within the profession will continue because for all its rhetoric about being a medical specialism like any other and all the drug company research and marketing to maintain the brain disease assertion, we are no wiser. No technical fixes have been found. Each new wonder drug brings with it new iatrogenic effects, which are life diminishing and sometimes life threatening. Madness like birth and death refuses to shake off its mysterious quality. And the mystery of madness is not the only tantalising question to consider. The ambit of psychiatry in the last hundred years extends far beyond what used to be called 'lunacy'. Speculations about how many more categories will be added to the next revision of the American Psychiatric Associations Diagnostic and Statistical Manual are rekindled every few years.

Recently at a conference I heard a very prestigious psychiatrist assert with great passion that it was vital to distinguish between mental disorder and social non-conformity. She echoed the APA's (American Psychiatric Association) own concern in this regard. But how do we actually make that distinction? With each and every form of madness, misery and badness being judged by their social consequences (what Scheff called 'residual rule breaking') there is no obvious logical or sociological distinction to be made.

Every psychiatric crisis is a social crisis and 'mental health law' is a misnomer. The social control of mental disorder is what legislation overwhelmingly deals with not mental health. The concerned psychiatrist at our conference warned of the danger of replaying the political role of psychiatry in the old Soviet Union. But why is it terrible to lock up political dissidents and turn them into salivating shuffling zombies but not terrible to do exactly the same to others, who also have broken no law but are called 'mentally disordered'? Clearly we cannot leave the business of mental health problems singularly to a profession whose leaders are unable to reflect honestly on their own regular political role and social context.

Contributors to this collection are drawn from a range of backgrounds and from very different social contexts. The user leaders contributions (Beresford and Wallcraft) highlight the long journey in front of those of us who wish to ensure that people experiencing mental illness will be supported in controlling their lives. Joan Rapaport illustrates the problematic treatment of relatives within the British mental health act, in which social workers play a major role side by side with psychiatrists.

All of the contributors explore central aspects of the psychosocial corrective to the bio-medical model and the assumption that new legislation necessarily marks progress. The reader will find much to think about in each chapter.

Undoubtedly the recurrent tension I noted at the start will keep throwing up new grounds for a psychosocial critique after the book is finished. This is a 2005 take from some interested authors on a long struggle.

David Pilgrim

Acknowledgements

We would like to thank all of the contributors to this book for the thoughtfulness with which they have approached the task of writing for this book.

Our thanks are due to Roxana Anghel who produced the final copy of the book, and has thus made our load more manageable, as well as to the Ashgate team responsible for its production.

We would like to thank each other for being generous in sharing ideas, supportive at every successive stage, and for completing the demanding task of editing this book while remaining good friends.

Shulamit Ramon and Janet E. Williams

Introduction

Janet E. Williams and Shulamit Ramon

This book was our response and challenge to the enduring status and domination of a bio-medical understanding and delivery of mental health services which, to quote from Roberto Mezzina's chapter, appears to many stakeholders 'superseded and anachronistic'. Worldwide there is an articulate challenge to this 'neo-positivist' illusion as well as alternative theories and practices; we have sought to give voice to this by inviting practitioners, academics and service users from Australia, Brazil, Italy, the UK, and USA to write from their standpoints in their area of expertise. They, like us, write not as critical theoreticians but with an active practical concern about the stigma and damage to individual's lives that this 'scientific' and diagnosis based approach brings. The style of writing reflects the differing cultural sources, but all challenge an unthinking reliance upon a simplistic scientific notion of scientific/research evidence. The chapters are theoretical, polemical at times, with a clear exposition of the values and politics of a psychosocial approach.

The title suggests an optimism that there is sufficient critical mass to challenge and make changes to this hegemonic paradigm. We are equally aware, and in fact illustrate in some of the chapters (Double, Healy and Renouf), that there have been such critical points in the past when new ideas and paradigm shifts have occurred. We present this collection with the intention of showing some of the history to this challenge, to illustrate trends, to elaborate upon movements still being shaped and to discuss theory with plenty of illustrations and case examples. We want this book to speak to a wide audience of service users and carers, theoreticians, policy makers, researchers, students and practitioners. The chapters are written with an enthusiasm and belief in the emancipation of service users, carers and practitioners; as well as in structural change alongside valuing the individual's subjective and narrative experience.

We have termed this way forward as 'psychosocial'. Though used before, we use it here to illustrate a paradigm in which both are integrated. The social includes the structural elements of society, such as social class, ethnicity, gender and sexual orientation, which affect not only the prevalence of poor mental health but the opportunities to access appropriate services, to be listened to, to make 'healthy' changes to the social and physical environment, to move out of social exclusion or to escape from violence. It also includes the impact of culture on mental health *and* illness. Psychological perspectives bring these ideas into both the subjective and intersubjective spheres, help with aetiology, and direct us to understand individual's and groups' experiences or narratives, the ways that people cope and make sense of their lives. However the danger of a purely psychological approach can be to pathologise, extending notions of illness ever wider by dint of our professional expertise fuelled by fear of risk taking, thus ignoring the breadth of 'normality' in society whether it be hearing voices, the extent of deprivation and poverty, or the incidence of women in abusive relationships.

The book is presented in four parts. The new and old paradigms are presented by the editors in Part One – Mental Health at the Crossroads – to contextualise the book and draw out the key elements of a psychosocial approach. Part Two – Contextualised Social Policy: Agenda and Priorities – demonstrates how the psychosocial approaches are shaped, promoted or hindered by policy and legislation; the confusion of ideas and competing influences which play a role in policy formation. Part Three – Paradigm Shift: Processes and Outcomes – considers the paradigm shift in more theoretical detail whilst Part Four – The Psychosocial: Experience and Practice – illustrates the policy and theory in practice.

Part One   Mental Health at the Crossroads

The first chapter, written by the editors, 'Towards a Conceptual Framework: The Meanings Attached to the Psychosocial, the Promise and the Problems', outlines the theoretical premise of the book and identifies issues discussed fully in the subsequent chapters. The 'psychosocial' is articulated and some contrasts made with other current models such as the bio-medical and the biopsychosocial. The psychosocial as used here denotes a demotion of the biological rather than a denial, and a subsequent questioning of the usefulness of bio-medical notions, such as 'diagnosis' and 'cure' in favour of terms that relate to people's lives and experience. For this reason the chapter begins with a case study in which the real lived issues such as depression are presented. The significance of the interrelationship between the social and psychological is explored to develop a more sophisticated understanding of each together. The case study provides different understandings and responses and in this way the 'existing hegemonic paradigm ... its un-usefulness – either/or conceptually, methodologically, ethically and in everyday intervention' (Mezzina) is revealed.

This leads to the extrapolation of the new perspective in which the user/patient relationship with the practitioner is highly significant; a relationship that is both more complex and profound than in physical medicine and which challenges traditional perspectives on professionalism. In line with emancipatory practices, which characterise the new psychosocial approach, this relationship is finely tuned to the power differentials, to the person's own life and becomes atypically 'hands on' in ways that rely upon the emotional/psychological availability of practitioners.

Part Two   Contextualised Social Policy: Agenda and Priorities

This section of the book takes some of the common psychosocial themes and explores their adoption or otherwise through policy making in three countries, the

UK, USA and Australia. These themes include integrated support, health promotion and prevention, social inclusion and quality of life issues through whole community support, sensitivity to ethnicity and culture, gender, sexual orientation as well as civil rights and the right to treatment. The authors show how the impact of political responses, from neo-liberal government to de-institutionalisation, are now associated with 'risk management' or 'risk aversion' in these countries and how this conflicts with the emergence of the voice of service users and the psychosocial approaches noted above. Both positions can be legislated for in different ways, but protection and control are given greater weight than the rights of service users. As demonstrated this is a contested field with considerable complexity due to the range of stakeholders, the lack of consensus about the balance between individual rights and community protection, different paradigms about mental distress and subsequently differing emphases on interventions.

Neil Foster's chapter starts this section by exploring how the concept of risk has taken on new, negative connotations, which have seriously affected policy making. He applies this to a case study, in three national contexts. Bill Healy and Noel Renouf consider the conflicting standpoints in an Australian context and then Pauline Prior addresses them in the UK, with reference to Europe.

Neil Foster takes risk as his starting point in the chapter entitled: 'Control, Citizenship and 'Risk' in Mental Health: Perspectives from UK, USA and Australia'. He uses a case study to illustrate how at the level of service provision citizenship, service entitlement and control/community protection are managed in practice through legal frameworks. The three societies have different legal frameworks but there is considerable convergence around a 'risk aversion' agenda, with an increased focus on managerialism. He argues that the mental health professional, subject to more bureaucratic surveillance is much less inclined towards therapeutic risk taking. This has meant that the care/control balance is the major focus for most mental health practitioners.

He points out the irony that concurrent with raised political expectations of public services and practitioners to manage risk has come a political challenge to, and subsequent erosion of, professional knowledge and expertise. He argues that risk has also become the eligibility factor for services so that those deemed 'low risk' are defined as 'less eligible'. He shows how the dominance of risk and rationing, following on from the wider political agenda, have served to exacerbate social exclusion while at the same time the user movement, requiring practitioners and government to enhance service users' rights, inclusion and services has been strengthened. The case study that follows is discussed in the policy and legal contexts each of the three countries in order to illustrate the tensions outlined above and the comparative differences.

Healy and Renouf in their chapter, 'Contextualised Social Policy: An Australian Perspective' provide an overview of influences and policy. Like Prior in the following chapter they pull out two competing themes or 'interests of progress' operating in the 'conflictual circumstances' influencing these changes. They identify these in the Australian context as care and community concern on the one hand whilst on the other competing definitions of what constitutes the system's preferred mode of intervention with identified service users, within the context of the competing paradigms of the bio-medical or the psychosocial.

The first National Mental Health Plan 1992 was constituted in order to improve services in response to de-institutionalisation. However the psychosocial interests embedded in it lost out to the seemingly more efficient medical interventions following a change of government and the subsequent neo-liberal reforms of welfare affecting working practices, reducing budgets. The second National Plan in 1998 reinstated the psychosocial aspects, reflecting World Health Organisation (WHO) guidance which stressed the burden of illness and that outcomes relate more to quality of life issues over levels of symptomology. They then outline the developments in their own State of Victoria using the same themes.

They go on to show how the fear of those supported by community services has not been dispelled by governments in Australia, but taken on board for political reasons and identified as a risk to be legislated for. They argue that the legislation has been counter productive because the introduction of compulsory treatment in the community – community treatment orders – damaged the work with service users through jeopardising the collaborative relationships between them which is key to recovery and effective shared assessment. Also this approach relies upon managing the illness rather than the quality of life and ignores civil rights. They state that the preoccupation with risk infects the whole culture of mental health work. This has brought about a greater focus on the medical aspects for mental health and very little attention to social care and social provision.

Prior gives a critique of current mental health policy in the UK from two similar contrasting and conflicting standpoints, one of rights and the other from risk and community protection, making links to similar debates within Europe. Within the UK she explores the 'modernisation' agenda since 1997, which has been introduced into all parts of government, welfare and health services. This is an agenda shared with the governments of most economically developed countries who have moved to community based mental health services with the effect, she says, of bringing them currently to a period of 'radical change'. She notes how mental health policy, unlike the rest of health policy also reflects changes to policy about crime, law and order. Prior considers that the combination of these changes has exacerbated the sense of risk. In parallel is the second trend, the slowly developing influence of the user movement which has grown in strength since the 1980s and which has aimed to increased citizenship. She gives many examples of how the Human Rights Act, introduced from the European Union since 1997, should be supporting the claims of service users.

The introduction of new Mental Health Act is likely to widen the scope of compulsory powers for enforced medication, following the Australian example. This has been criticised by almost all stakeholder as diminishing civil rights and because it is likely to be unworkable. This challenge to civil rights, mitigates against the worker/user relationship outlined as crucial in a psychosocial approach, as discussed by Foster, Healy and Renouf above, as well as by Ramon, Williams and in Wallcrafts's chapter on Recovery.

Part Three   Paradigm Shift: Process and Outcomes

This section of the book provides theoretical and historical perspectives on the paradigm shifts inherent in the development of psychosocial approaches and suggestions for ways forward. The field is contested and this is reflected in the authors' contributions which bring differing emphases along the psychosocial spectrum. The first theme, written in two complementary chapters by two psychiatrists illustrates this. The first half, written by Duncan Double starts with a critical discussion of the more traditional biopsychosocial model whilst Roberto Mezzina's outlines a psychosocial service in a more overtly social and political way. These are followed by Eduardo Vasconcelos' account from a global structural perspective in which he explains the global impact upon the development of a psychosocial service in a less economically developed, but huge country – Brazil. The section is completed by a return to the individual, the service user as citizen and stakeholder in the development of psychosocial perspectives. Peter Beresford, in a socially orientated chapter discusses the psychosocial from a service users perspective and develops another theme common to this book, the impact of the medical hegemony of the bio-medical model.

Duncan Double's chapter, 'Paradigm Shift in Psychiatry', is in two complementary parts. These in different ways provide some history of the development of paradigms. Double's contribution provides a history of the biopsychosocial model and the progress which it represented. Mezzina on the other hand takes the psychosocial from a much more socio/political standpoint and provides the elements of a new paradigm which is more dependent on the social and in particular the requisites for the transfer from institutionalisation to de-institutionalisation. He also describes a service which is fully integrated with the locality in all its parts and reflects a 'hands on' approach.

Both authors are critical of the bio-medical model as reductionist and Double lays out the history of alternative approaches such as the biopsychosocial, the retrenchment into the neurobiological and its ascendancy as a reaction by orthodox psychiatry, to the anti-psychiatric movement in the 1970s. He argues that in the USA psychiatry is no longer as open to alternatives as once it was and its professional standing is now contingent upon the bio-medical model; he questions whether this in now an impregnable position. To answer this he deconstructs the bio-medical paradigm in terms of the social and theoretical elements it contains and considers how these can be upturned in order that this trend be reversed and a return made to a more appropriate paradigm, the biopsychosocial.

Double emphasises a number of points that are also significant in the psychosocial model including a concern with: the life story of the individual; meaningful existence as more significant for mental health than brain chemistry; and human action as complex and ultimately unpredictable. However, he is rightly critical of simplistic explanations of causation or social deviance as evidence for a complex psychological phenomenon, though this latter point is developed further in Neil Foster's chapter and by David Pilgrim in the forward.

The parallel part of this section on paradigm shifts comes from Roberto Mezzina who reflects upon the experience of, and current practice within, the 'democratic psychiatry' movement in Italy, and Trieste in particular. He makes the point that, despite de-institutionalisation, the rationale of the asylum usually remains in community services through the use of coercion and exclusion. In parallel, as the forms of treatment and locus extend so does the pathologisation and medicalisation of the 'normal'.

He is optimistic of a paradigm shift, away from a 'treating illness model', to one which emphasises a response to real and tangible needs, including the psychological and highly subjective, in a very personal journey of recovery. With this as the guiding principle he illustrates a series of processes and aims and the corresponding 'paradigm shifts' needed. He warns against selectivity and fragmentation by speciality of services which have the effect of excluding some service users over time and instead calls for a service which 'shoulders the burden' by being a 'service for life'. He calls for a service which works with service users as citizens and which is fully engaged with all the components of people's geographical community and social networks, their subjectivities and 'lived' time; in other words all dimensions of daily lives.

Eduardo Vasconcelos writes about Brazil in his chapter called 'Structural Issues Underpinning Mental Health Care and Psychosocial Approaches in Developing Countries: The Brazilian Case'. Starting from the world stage, he provides a framework for making cross-national comparisons of mental health services in less economically developed countries. This framework is used to review the psychiatric reforms in Brazil in terms of a psychosocial approach. It is clear from this chapter that such comparison, or evaluation of service development, needs to take account of the social and structural context as well as globalisation and international financial directives for structural adjustment such as fiscal crises, increasing poverty and social violence. Mental health provisions and the model of choice in the development process have to be reviewed in the light of these influences to the political and social fabric of the society which is more unstable than more economically developed countries.

He tracks the process of change from a revolutionary wave and widespread, general demands for the realization of rights, including help with mental health problems. Such social and demographic changes have the potential to lessen support as stable and hierarchical cultural structures breakdown. These were very supportive of people with mental health problems in Brazil and offered a better prognosis for recovery than later when these were substituted by neo-liberal welfare services. He takes the parameters for a psychosocial approach, with many features similar to those outlined in Mezzina's chapter, illustrating how these have fared in the development of Brazil and its mental health services.

Peter Beresford's is the concluding chapter in this section on paradigm changes. He starts from the perspective of the service user. His particular focus is epistemology, the 'knowledge sources' that comes from them and other less well represented stakeholders, and the impact that these can have on their participation in the development of mental health' ideas and praxis. He deconstructs the social model and outlines in detail a more complex and sophisticated version which deals with the structural without ignoring agency taking on board the individual and psychological aspects in a non-pathologising way in line with the psychosocial approach being promoted in this book. The question of care is moved to one of rights in line with a citizenship model of using services.

Part Four   The Psychosocial: Experience and Practice

This section of the book applies the psychosocial approach to a number of contemporary themes and practice areas in mental health and starts with two chapters based on service user's perspectives, the themes of recovery by Jan Wallcraft and self-help and mutual support by Carol Munn-Giddings and Thomasina Borkman. These chapters outline in some detail the core features of practice that have emerged from the user movement since the 1980s. A chapter on the informal caring experience by Joan Rapaport, follows, then chapters on trauma (Janet E. Williams), mental health promotion (Shulamit Ramon), the psychosocial in an educational context (Julia Jones and Catherine Gamble) and spirituality (Phil Barker and Poppy Buchanan-Barker).

Jan Wallcraft describes the 'recovery paradigm' as a unifying factor in a broad alliance between psychosocial professionals and academics, the voluntary sector and the service user movement. Its origins lie in the user movements coming primarily from the USA and the UK and as a paradigm it incorporates both a structural perspective, attention to the power differentials within professional/user relations as well individual subjectivity in terms of their own aims for 'recovery' and their lives. She explains its meaning as a framework, still contested and developing, that should replace notions of cure and rehabilitation because it is a fundamentally different way of taking account of mental health problems and the persons who experience it. In the recovery model, 'getting better' is not equated with medical ideas of cure and challenges the routine of rehabilitation. Hope is very significant as it relates to the individual's own narrative and aims. Recovery presents a fundamental challenge to the bio-medical models but acknowledging the power of the latter she is careful to warn against it being incorporated, at the expense of its true complexity and aims. Wallcraft shows how despite a growing consensus even in groups who were previously against it in the USA, it risks being used to the detriment of the social and psychological needs of service users if it is incorporated into the whole machinery of the bio-medical industry of research, policy and funding related to physical treatments.

The chapter, 'Self-Help/Mutual Aid as a Psychosocial Phenomenon' by Carol Munn-Giddings and Thomasina Borkman outlines long existing, practical alternatives to services based upon traditional scientific approaches, in the form of mutual support groups and reciprocal forms of self-help. The authors provide historical perspectives to these developments, contrasting the UK and the USA. Though these forms of support are widespread they are not usually mainstream so have not been widely researched and are not yet fully recognized. Mutual aid is based upon the principle of a user led service and should not be confused or conflated with traditional self-help or other therapeutically organized groups or activities.

They place self-help/mutual aid firmly within a social and political context though it is grounded in the experiential and subjective; the lived experience of service users. The forums are led and controlled by service users and provide a group presence of peers for those who want to understand their experiences better (consciousness raising) and in relation to collective knowledge, described by Borkman as 'disciplined subjectivity'. This process also offers service users the opportunity to work collectively for change and improvements in services. From the research they conclude that the relationship between these 'informal groups' and formal services has to be negotiated but the presence of the former produces more discerning and assertive service users, making better use of services. On the back of these developments have come local and national policy changes and in places some change to traditional services.

A complementary chapter to this is from Joan Rapaport entitled 'The Informal Caring Experience: Issues and Dilemmas'. Rapaport suggests that we are still lacking a body of research into the needs and roles of carers and there has not been an overarching theoretical framework or set of governing principles to shape its development. In this chapter she takes the carer's perspective in relation to their own needs but also makes the case for the benefits to service users when this is done appropriately with full awareness of the tensions and potential dilemmas. Rapaport also proposes that together the carer and the Approved Social Worker (the ASW, the UK social worker who is required by law to look for the least restrictive alternatives when compulsory treatment is being considered) can together combat undue medical pressure for admission to hospital.

She provides a detailed policy overview of their position, difficulties in practice that can arise from their inclusion, especially in the process of compulsory hospital admissions since in the UK they potentially have as much power as the other nominated person, the ASW. She highlights how they can be involved in service user care planning as well as in the more recent UK policy which entitles them to an assessment of their own needs quite separately from that of the service users'. Carers' views, she argues, should also figure in the considerations of risk since they have been the victims of well publicised homicides.

The chapter 'Living with Trauma' (Janet E. Williams) takes a term that is now being used more frequently in mental health; whether it be to understand those who have experienced child sexual abuse (CSA), post traumatic stress, war or torture. It is argued that understanding trauma is an aide to understanding the huge impact of the psychological and social processes on all aspects of everyday life. Since the specialist mental health services are populated by people who have experienced trauma it is essential to have a comprehensive understanding. Diagnoses of depression, anxiety, borderline personality disorder often hide the lived experiences of trauma, some of which continue in adult form in terms of abusive relationships, self-harm, flashbacks and low self esteem. The psychological theory is analysed with some discussion about how this can be used constructively, avoiding pathologising coping mechanisms which were essential for survival. The social impact of CSA is also discussed, its intrusion into achieving in school, making friends, social exclusion, awareness of difference and later on employment prospects, confidence and assertiveness in relationships and self esteem. These are teased out in a case study which also illustrates the continued powerlessness of some women, and survivors in the mental health system.

A further case study is explored in relation to an asylum seeker. Again the starting point is not pathology, but the need to look at social difficulties; social exclusion, racism and the attitudes of those in services they access which can be more problematic and destructive than the trauma they experienced. Psychological difficulties may be coped with in ways that are culturally appropriate, which is not to avoid providing help but not to conclude that people from all cultures want the same thing. The psychosocial approach presented again draws heavily on mutuality, community activity, cultural appropriateness and reciprocity in a model that relates closely to the philosophy in the recovery model.

In the chapter 'Unpacking Mental Health Promotion' Shulamit Ramon begins by providing conceptual clarity about the terminology associated with differing models of mental health promotion and considers its political significance using some cross national comparisons to illustrate these aspects. 'Well being' is the preferred term, which removes mental health promotion from the dominant paradigm of medicine to a social context, and it is discussed as a range of dimensions and as a process, in which the individual may define themselves. It thus becomes a more complex concept than the more familiar ones of absence of illness or disease and raises questions about the meaning of the universal term, mental ill health. It is also discussed in relation to risk as it is currently conceptualised in terms of avoidance, also education and protection which she argues are very different in mental health compared with physical health. This means that mental health promotion requires a different understanding, policy, strategy, methods, and implementation because there is a complex interaction between biological, psychological and social factors. In contrast health promotion in the public health model tends to imply personal responsibility without regard for those who are not always in a position to shoulder it and it ignores the social context of behaviours. The psychosocial approach in this chapter reflects the notions of prevention, education and protection, which are similar to the recovery model outlined in Jan Wallcraft's chapter.

Thus mental health promotion is complex and if it is to have meaning needs to face some of the underlying causes which include social exclusion, oppression and structural factors. Work on a community and societal level is needed if it is to be truly preventative rather than intervening once problems emerge. Examples from the Netherlands as well as the UK are provided to illustrate this.

The following chapter, 'Re-introducing the Psychosocial in Training, Education and Research' by Julia Jones and Catherine Gamble describes the history and development of behavioural psychosocial approaches, used recently to manage the symptoms of those with severe and enduring mental health problems, and the training provided. Though these approaches have had the rhetoric of a holistic approach there has been some criticism that these interventions have used a bio-medical management approach. In this chapter the authors outline how these should take account of the service user agendas of rights, citizenship and collaboration.

Initially the training was only delivered to community psychiatric nurses, to help reduce relapses with those with diagnosis of schizophrenia. The aim was to increase knowledge and skills, to challenge pessimistic assumptions about schizophrenia and thus reduce the reliance on medication and hospital to manage symptoms. Now the training focuses upon psychosocial factors as well as the more traditional ones, including recovery, individualized, tailor made self-help methods, such as the normalization of experiences, spirituality and complementary therapies. The aims are to help users feel more empowered, valued and able to function within society. The training approach is also designed to link in supervisors and managers and users' expertise which is incorporated into curriculum development, teaching and supervision. The components of the training include assessment, medication, psychological management of psychosis and early intervention, family needs and intervention in which very practical and psychosocial interventions are used such as making sense and managing voices. These approaches are then demonstrated through a full discussion and analysis of a case study in which the issues and potential problems and interventions are outlined.

The last contribution to the book which completes Part Four, 'The Psychosocial: Experience Practise' is entitled 'Spirituality and Mental Health: An Integrative Dimension' written by Phil Barker and Poppy Buchanan-Barker. This brings the reader to another definition of mental health that has been hinted at by other contributions, that of 'meaning making' 'subjectivities' 'narratives', in the lives of individuals experiencing the confusions of mental distress. This chapter starts there, not with policy, or professional language but with something that is common to everyone, whether recognised or not – spiritual wellbeing. This topic and the chapter is not about information but is intended to be thought provoking; as the authors say spirituality is about experience not words. They explore how we find 'self' whatever that might be and 'self-knowledge' as a perpetual journey to call into our awareness of being. However their approach is not a quest as such but about using what we have as we live it. This is not the usual language of mental health texts or practice and as such it may trigger resistance, especially for its assumed relationship with organized religion.

They make the point, as others have that though we have more and more categories of mental illness and seemingly more explanations this does not address the problem that everyone has of giving meaning to their lives and the events which unfold. It is in this sense that spirituality contributes as one avenue for constructing meaning. However, it goes beyond the individual since this approach is a challenge as it sidesteps the systems and codes of psychiatry, the diagnoses, the idea of people as no more than brain function, genes and chemistry. Equally their focus on spirituality challenges psychotherapy, though it can be the starting point for discovering it. It also finds 'echoes in poetry, literature, opera and the visual arts; if not also magic, ritual and humankind's primeval relationship to time and place'. Thus spirituality brings the professionals back to what they don't know, to their openness, humility and even ignorance. This returns to one of the fundamental structures of the psychosocial, the new forms of relationships and alliances between professionals and service users.

In summary we believe the text offers a wide ranging psychosocial framework which can compete as a viable alternative to the more traditional bio-medical model and in all spheres be they experiential, conceptual, policy, practice and research within the field of mental health.

Part One
Mental Health at the Crossroads

Chapter 1

Towards a Conceptual Framework: The Meanings attached to the Psychosocial, the Promise and the Problems

Shulamit Ramon and Janet E. Williams

Alice is a good looking woman in her early 30s, who has given recently birth to her second child, and is 'mildly' depressed. In conversation with the health visitor she lists the reasons why she should not be depressed, weepy and lethargic, ending the list by saying 'I know that I am ungrateful for all that I have got and undeserving of it, but I still am depressed'. She described her lack of joy in having the new baby, in being with the older child (now five-years-old), of finding it increasingly difficult to get up in the morning, to get the children dressed, the house in order, of only wanting to stay in bed covered by a blanket, on her own, of being unresponsive to her partner's wishes and needs, of finding what people talk about too trivial and of no relevance to her life. She is also worried about being a good enough mother and cannot imagine herself going back to work.

She did not experience depression after the birth of her first child, has a satisfying – but demanding – job to go back to, a supportive but weary and easily irritable partner, has no friends in the neighbourhood to which they have moved six months ago.

It would be easy to prescribe her antidepressants and tell her she will feel much better when the tablets will kick in within three weeks. Such a response will be perceived as a confirmation that the pregnancy and birth have led to a chemical imbalance, corrected by the drugs. This would leave untouched the issues of why has this reaction did not take place after the first birth, her fears for the future, the apparent isolation, her fragility, or the fact that the 'mild' depression is experienced by her, her partner – and no doubt her children too – as a very unhappy state to be in.

If, instead, Alice would be given access to a help line volunteer, a weekly group of women at different stages of postnatal depression to join, to which a crèche is attached, with the option to take the antidepressants or not, she may have as a result a support network, an opportunity to discuss her issues within an empathic setting, listen to the issues and solutions raised by others, and make a much more informed decision as to whether she needs medication, counselling, to go back to a half-time post and when, what helps her when weepy, and perhaps increase the enjoyable elements of her life.

At present Alice is much more likely to be given only antidepressants. It is a matter of luck whether her GP will know of a help line, whether s/he will even consider the usefulness of such an alternative, or whether the health visitor will raise this possibility with her and her GP.

A paradigm shift in the context of mental health is in existence when we begin to doubt whether the usefulness of the existing hegemonic paradigm is over taken by its un-usefulness – either/or conceptually, methodologically, ethically, and in everyday intervention. The harm seems to outweigh the benefit attributed to such an approach; when central planks of the issues at stake are not taken into account – or denied attention – by that hegemonic paradigm according to major stakeholders; the beginning of an alternative perspective is delineated.

We would be arguing in this book that indeed we have reached this state of doubt concerning the hegemonic model of mental health, namely the 'medical' model, or more correctly the biochemical model of mental illness. The issues denied prominence and due attention form a long list, including themes such as:

- The social context and its variables
- Health as distinct from the absence of illness
- The psychological layer as an etiological factor, including the impact of abuse
- Power relationships and their impact within the mental health system and in its wider social context
- Recovery as a realistic option for people with psychosis.

The continuous invention of new types of medication, some with fewer side effects than the previous generation and hence more effective in suppressing symptoms and enabling people to lead a more ordinary life, is presented as the proof that the biochemical model is working well and should not be discarded.

No one would wish to deny relief to people who suffer relief from pain. Yet it needs to be asked at what cost to them – and to the rest of us – is this relief obtained. Is it long lasting? Have the alternatives been given a fair trial? If Alice would take the medication prescribed would she be able to stop taking it at the end of the period prescribed by her doctor, or would she become dependent on it?

Why, despite these achievements, more and more people – lay and professionals alike – are raising their doubts as to the validity and effectiveness of the medical model (Rogers, Pilgrim and Lacey, 1993; Ramon, 2003)?

In typical relationships between doctors and patients or nurses and patients, the latter are often grateful for the professional intervention offered by the first. Yet fewer of those using mental health services express such gratitude. When asked, users would indicate that they have met good and bad practitioners; highlighting that the difference between the two is not about their professional ability but whether they treated the user as a person, whether they felt respected, cared for and attended to as a human being. This response, especially expressed in the context of in-patient facilities, reflects some of the key differences between medicine and psychiatry. Users of mental health services can easily be seen as needy of, or greedy for, attention, due to being in turmoil, feeling a failure and being rejected by others, especially when in crisis. They therefore seek to be compensated for the above in the contact with professionals, but often feel rebuffed. While some of the difficulties in the relationships are related to lack of enough workers able to provide good enough attention, it is also true that medicine – of which psychiatry is a branch – trains professionals who focus on the part that needs to be cured, while being polite and courteous. Being polite and courteous is insufficient in terms of the type of attention the sufferer from mental distress or illness wishes for and requires. This way of relating to people implies that professionalism is not about a distanced, 'hands off' approach, but instead requires emotional closeness, a 'hands on' approach, and the demonstration of interest in those everyday affairs which matter to the service user. Alice felt truly relived when the health visitor asked her to tell her in detail about getting up in the morning and preparing the children for the new day, and even seemed genuinely interested in what she had to tell. It was the first time that a professional showed an interest in what she found particularly difficult, but could not bring herself to discuss as it was 'so trivial', and she was sure none of the professionals would be interested.

Providing satisfactory care in mental health is a mentally and psychologically demanding activity, one which requires considerable time, continuity and hence a sufficient number of sufficiently qualified people to carry it through adequately. The 'hands on' approach which enables the client to get on with her/his life, the shortening of the distance between professionals and users, and the demonstrable *emotional availability* of the worker is what marks good psychosocial professionalism from the traditional model of practising psychiatry.

Although low in technological costs, mental health services are bound to be financially expensive because they are labour intensive, and will need to be largely met through public sector funding. Nevertheless, there are significant differences as to the cost of different forms of interventions and policies, with hospital care being the more costly setting.

The critique of the medical model in the context of mental health has focused on its denial of the existence of the impact of the social context in leading to mental distress, in interacting with any biological or psychological intervention, and therefore in impacting on recovery too. This critique is not new; its hay day dating back to the 1960–1980s. The core of that critique has been since accepted as valid, yet most of it has been neatly ignored by the protagonists of the medical model and those circles impacted by them. This attests to the power of the medical model within and outside the mental health system, and the relative lack of power of the protagonists of the critique. It also reflects the degree of discomfort this critique causes to those who are in the position of acting upon it.

For example, we are witnessing now the introduction of mental health teams to primary care, staffed by nurses with skills in brief psychological interventions, for which there is a convincing evidence base of the likely benefit to the many people approaching primary care presenting the first signs of depression and other types of minor mental illnesses (Armstrong, 1995). Likewise early psychosocial intervention in psychosis is proving to be a valuable intervention (Jackson and Farmer, 1998, and chapter 11 by Jones and Gamble in this text), as are attempts to work within a psycho-educational model with families (Falloon and Fadden, 1992).

This new way of working reflects the recognition of the value of psychological interventions, as distinct from – though not in opposition to – the medical model. It attests to the acceptance that medication for these types of difficulties is, at best, of limited value because it does not enable the person to develop better problem solving and coping strategies, but instead fosters a denial of the implications of the symptoms and their meaning in the person's context.

Yet the same approach to mental health in primary care is taken regardless of whether the practice is based in a run down or a posh area; ignoring the level of poverty, isolation, and socio-economic deprivation to be found in a poor area to which clients return from the brief intervention.

A new national initiative regarding the reduction of domestic violence, because of its damage to the mental health of women and children, started in 2002, yet the connection between domestic violence, minor and major mental illness was not made and the most recent interventions for the latter are not informed by the former.

No attempt is made to take account of these structural factors and handle their impact as appropriate to different populations, reflecting the fragmentation between psychological and social perspectives, and the fragmentation in the level of acceptability of each of those approaches within the medical establishment. Existing evidence of the usefulness of individual and group social work intervention in primary care, pioneered in the UK in the 1960s and 1970s, has been ignored (Knight, 1978; Brewer and Lait, 1982), highlighting the selective use of existing evidence in favour of approaches which discomfort the protagonists of the medical model as little as possible, aimed at reducing pressure on GPs above all other objectives.

Simultaneously we have seen the revival of interest in mental health promotion and formulation of policies related to it, though without the necessary funding for their implementation, in a number of countries, such as Britain and Australia, for reasons explained in the chapters on contextualized social policy and the chapter on mental health promotion. On the one hand these provide a blueprint for the promotion of mental health in the context of reducing discrimination and social exclusion (see the British National Service Framework for Mental Health, DoH 1999). Schools and the workplace are cited as the sites of promising such interventions. On the other hand these policies extend the remit of psychiatry, and its social control mandate, even further than is the case presently. This duality of a liberating force, which can also be oppressive, is inherent within the mental health system, and is not unique to its mental health promotion component (Rose and Miller, 1986; Pilgrim and Rogers, 1999).

The inclusion of mental health promotion in the context of discrimination and exclusion, the increased focus on the value of employment, and the belief in the ability to work of people with long term mental ill health are some of the signs that at long last the critique of the medical model is finding its way into the official platform of the priorities to be achieved in – and by – the mental health system. The official platform has been composed in all Western countries with the collaboration of all mental health disciplines, as well as that of users and carers, led by psychiatrists able to put together the psychological and the social perspectives side by side with a version of the medical model. Whether this version has *coherence*, and whether there is coherence in separating out the social from the psychological, is one of the issues to be explored in this book. The shift in the official platform reflects the shift in the paradigm which underlined the mental health system up to this point in time.

We, and all of the contributors to this volume, would wish to argue that the split between the social and the psychological risks would turn the achievement of putting the two on the policy map into an empty victory, which would reinforce the denial of the interactive relationships between these two dimensions by the purists of the medical model.

Some of us – notably Duncan Double – are wishing to reconstruct the biopsychological model, initially proposed by the German-Jewish, American, psychiatrist Adolph Meyer in the early part of the 20th century. Arguing that biology plays a part in mental distress, illness and health seems commonsensical for creatures rooted within a body, as we all are. Yet in the history of the medical model giving priority to biology has meant the denial of all else as of primary importance, a position the contributors to this book would disagree with for reasons outlined in a number of the chapters, ranging from the chapter on risk, through the chapters on self-defining scenarios and the recovery narrative, to the chapters on spirituality, self-help, and trauma. As a result, few of the authors to this collection would wish to see the biological dimension given the same priority as the social and psychological ones, but the argument for such a perspective will be outlined in this collection, enabling the reader to make his/her own judgement as to its viability. However, it is important to note that contributors to this book differ among themselves in the focus on the social vs. the focus on the psychological.

This chequered, evolving, recent history of the psychosocial approach highlights its complexity and the potential for more than one meaning being attached to it, and therefore more than one approach to its application at the conceptual, methodological and practice layers. This text aims at unravelling this complexity at the different levels.

One of the arguments for putting the biological perspective on unequal footing to the psychosocial approach is the place of *health* within the past and current 'mental health' system. Although titled mental health the latter concept has been defined within the medical model only as the absence of disease and illness. It was left to the psychosocial approach protagonists to give health meanings of its own, which range from the psychoanalytic definition of the *ability to love and work* to *the achievement of the sense of coherence*.

Equally the lack of distinction between distress, illness, and disease within psychiatry, where mainly *quantitative* differences in severity of symptoms are recognized through the use of the terms minor and severe mental illness, with an ever increasing number of diagnoses listed in the different versions of the American Diagnostic Statistical Manual (DSM) and the West European Indicators of Classified Diagnoses (ICD10), demonstrating this lack of conceptual refinement. The readiness to view any symptom as the reflection of an illness/disease highlights not only the over-determination of considering pathology to the exclusion of health, but also of the exclusion of human resilience, strength, and protective factors from the conceptual paradigm and the intervention strategy.

Thus the view of risk within the medical model is one preoccupied with *risk avoidance*, whereas in the psychosocial approach the potential exists for *risk taking*, if not necessarily a reality which welcomes the latter in mental health services and the thinking about users and carers, as Neil Foster's comparative chapter illustrates.

Risk has indeed become a dominant feature of late modern societies (Beck, 1992; Rose, 1999), for reasons related to the inherent uncertainty of social and personal life/living within such societies.

Psychiatry has been politically and culturally pressurized into accepting risk avoidance at the top of its practice agenda, without mounting any credible overt opposition to this pressure. Chinks in this overall position can be detected in everyday practice where personal and team discretion is utilized, but also more recently in the multidisciplinary opposition to the newly proposed British Mental Health Act in which it would become possible to detain people with the diagnosis of antisocial personality disorder without a deterioration in their mental state for preventive purposes. The objections are partly related to human rights principles, turning hospitalization into incarceration, doubting the therapeutic value of such a hospitalization. They also relate to the fear of an over-sweeping umbrella of risk avoidance which takes away the professional discretionary balancing decision-making function between risk avoidance and risk taking anchored within the psychosocial context of an individual.

The psychosocial approach incorporates the view of the *life cycle* as a central dimension within mental health thinking and acting. The significance of the life cycle lies in identifying common human conditions and events as likely to lead to common mental responses, including crisis, breakdown, copying, problem solving, and the potential for recovery. While the meaning attached to specific events throughout the life cycle would vary according to culture and socio-economic factors, such as *gender* and *ethnicity*, the universality of the life cycle itself enables us to learn from the particular to the general and vice versa.

Equally the recognition of the occurrence of mental health crises related to universal life events helps to reduce the stigma attached to such a crisis.

Traumas have also become a hallmark of late modernity, be they located in intimate relationships (child sexual abuse, domestic violence), in the wider social context (war, interethnic conflict) or due to natural and ecological disasters (earthquakes, chemical poisoning), and the toll of the ever increasing number of road accidents. We therefore need to understand better reactions to these events, the role played by vulnerability from the past, as much as the role played by psychological and social factors in the present. Such an understanding would enable us firstly, to include trauma within the diagnostic process, from which it is presently excluded. Secondly, taking such a perspective questions the validity of some diagnostic categories, notably personality disorder, where trauma, depression and socially unacceptable behaviour co-exist (Castillo, 2003). Thirdly a more holistic approach to trauma may lead us as a collective to more preventive efforts/programmes.

New Knowledge

Biological science, inclusive of medicine and psychiatry, continues to generate newly codified knowledge. The genes map is the latest such innovation, whose value to the field of mental health and illness is yet to be explored in a significant way. This type of knowledge does not seem to have at present legitimate space for the knowledge gained through tapping the direct, subjective and inter-subjective, experience of users of mental health services, lay and professional people. It continues to be based solely on natural science logic and methods, uninfluenced by most of what has been learned throughout the 20th century as to the narrowness and distortion of this type of knowledge when applied to mental health and illness.

Psychological and social knowledge, as interpreted by social scientists, has developed in parallel. This state of affairs is ironical in a context in which the patient/client/user is the main invaluable source of information. These interpretations depend to a considerable extent on the conceptual and ideological frameworks of their creators and protagonists.

Evidence

In parallel we have witnessed the attempts to correct these biased types knowledge by introducing a third category, derived from the experience of users (Ramon, 2003) and carers (Jones, 2001). These two groups are perceived as having expert knowledge of mental illness and health, as well as of services, which has been hitherto rejected, invalidated and/or neglected by professionals and scientists alike. The way through which this knowledge is tapped into is important in order to prevent its premature interpretation and codification by qualified researchers/social scientists and professionals. Some attempts have been made to enable *professionals* to reflect on their subjective and inter-subjective experience as an additional, complimentary, layer of knowledge (Winter *et al.*, 1999).

These have highlighted that the professionals grapple with basic existential issues not unlike those identified as clients – guilt, self worth, owe at the loss experienced by patients, and difficulties to come to terms with their own losses, how to express and how to receive empathy and praise.

The only parallel attempt to do so with lay people appears in fiction. Fiction, however, is a non-systematic tool, which can offer identification and catharsis, but not the systematic working through which good research, good professional supervision (and psychotherapy), can provide.

Engaging user researchers in this process reinforces the readiness to recall experience less mediated by social desirability, while increasing the process of empowerment for both the researchers and those being researched. This type of knowledge can challenge as well as corroborate knowledge acquired through other modes/forms, a task presently at its infancy.

Engaging users as evaluators of the work carried out with them is another facet of this type of evidence (Rose, 2001; Ramon, 2003), and is exemplified in Jones and Gamble's chapter.

This type of knowledge informs most of the chapters in this collection, such as the chapters on self-help, self defined scenarios, recovery, trauma, policy, and spirituality. It informs the underlying critical approach to traditional perspectives of mental illness and health and the search for an alternative psychosocial perspective, in evidence in all chapters,

Implications for Training

Introducing a new, or renewed, framework to a large multidisciplinary group of qualified and unqualified workers inevitably requires a re-appraisal of their training. A process of unlearning and relearning becomes imperative at the attitudinal, conceptual, methodological, and practice levels. Most qualified professionals find such a re-appraisal an upheaval, as it implies criticism of their previous state of professional being (Ramon, 1992). Yet it is possible through the allure of the new, in terms of increased and improved knowledge to bring professionals to learn new knowledge and skills. It is more difficult to change their value base. In many ways it is easier to change the framework unqualified workers bring with them than it is to change that of qualified workers, as the investment in the old is not that high for the first group.

The implications for training are outlined in the chapters on (Jones and Gamble), trauma and recovery.

What's in the Name, In-elegant as it is?

The term *psychosocial* is widely used by different camps – from those practising psychoanalysis to those practising cognitive behavioural approaches – to denote the combination of the psychological with the social, but is not found in any ordinary dictionary. It has been the hallmark of social work since the 1950s, when it was coined by Helen Perlman in conjunction with her problem solving approach to working with individuals and families (Perlman, 1957; Horobin, 1985).

The Promise

We believe that the application of the psychosocial approach would improve our state of understanding people experiencing mental distress and illness, the distress and illness themselves and mental health. Such an articulated understanding would enable us to improve the range of interventions on offer and their content, as highlighted in each of the chapters of this book.

The current state of knowledge enables us to state that the promise is not merely a belief, but one to which considerable evidence is attached, as reflected in each chapter within this book. Moreover, the focus on the psychosocial approach enables new forms of knowledge and of evidence to come to the fore, as highlighted in the chapters on trauma, recovery, self-defined scenarios, spirituality and mental health promotion.

We hope the readers will find the book stimulating and enjoyable.

References

Armstrong, L.C. (1995), *Mental Health Issues in Primary Care, A Practical Guide*, Macmillan, Basingstoke.

Beck, U. (1992), *The Risk Society: Towards a New Modernity*, Sage, London.

Brewer, A. and Lait, J. (1982), *Can Social Work Survive?*, Routledge, London.

Castillo, H. (2003), *Personality Disorder: Temperament or Trauma?*, Jessica Kingsley, London.

Department of Health (1999), *National Service Framework for Mental Health: Modern Standards and Service Models*, HMSO.

Falloon, I. and Fadden, G. (1992), 'Crisis intervention and intensive care for acute episodes: Creating an asylum at home', in: Falloon, I. (ed.), *Integrated Mental Health Care*, Cambridge University Press, Cambridge.

Horobin, G. (1985), *Responding to Mental Illness. Research Highlights in Social Work II*, Kogan Page, London.

Jackson, C. and Farmer, A. (1998), 'Early Intervention in Psychosis', *Journal of Mental Health*, 7, 2, 157-164.

Jones, D. (2001), *Myths, Madness and the Family: The Impact of Mental Illness on Families*, Macmillan, Basingstoke.

Knight, C. (1978), *Neighbourhood Groups*, Family Service Unit, London.

Perlman, H. (1957), *Social Casework*, University of Chicago Press, Chicago.

Pilgrim, D. and Rogers, A. (1999), *A Sociology of Mental Health and Illness*, The Open University, Buckingham, 2nd edition.

Ramon, S. (1992), 'The workers' perspective: Living with ambiguity, ambivalence and challenge', in: Ramon, S. (ed.), *Psychiatric Hospital Closure: Myths and Realities*, Chapman Hall, London, 85-119.

Ramon, S. (ed.) (2003), *Users Researching Health and Social Care*, Venture Press, Birmingham.

Rogers, A., Pilgrim, D. and Lacey, R. (1993), *Experiencing Psychiatry*, Mind Macmillan, Basingstoke.

Rose, D. (2001), *Users Voices*, Sainsbury Centre for Mental Health, London.

Rose, N. and Miller, P. (eds) (1986), *The Power in Psychiatry*, Polity Press, Cambridge.

Rose, N. (1999), *Powers of Freedom: Reframing Political Thought*, Cambridge University Press, Cambridge.

Winter, R., Buck, A. and Sobiechowska, P. (1999), *Professional Experience and The Investigative Imagination: The Art of Reflective Writing*, Routledge, London.

Part Two
Contextualised Social Policy:
Agenda and Priorities

Chapter 2

Control, Citizenship and 'Risk' in Mental Health: Perspectives from UK, USA and Australia

Neil Foster

Neil Foster is a community mental health manager in the UK and also an Approved social worker (ASW) under the Mental Health Act (1983). In the UK the approved social worker has a pivotal role in conjunction with medical professionals in the application of powers of compulsory admission to hospital. In this chapter Neil seeks to examine some of the mechanisms available to professionals in managing mental health risks in the community in three societies which exhibit a preoccupation with risk from professional and organisational points of view and where specific forms of legal control have evolved to secure compliance and satisfy growing public and political concerns. A comparative approach is adopted by using a case study/scenario which highlights how the law and service entitlements may interact in practice as events unfold, and how professional practices which enhance or inhibit citizenship entitlements are located within contrasting legal frameworks. In recent years in all three societies there has been a noticeable convergence of service forms and configurations in response to neo-liberal economic and welfare reforms, the political dominance of 'risk aversive' agendas, the challenges of de-institutionalisation and the increasing professional and managerial focus on what does and what does not work in community mental health. Rarely is 'best evidence' easily uncovered in this field, neither is it unproblematic to assume that consensus is easily reached as to what would constitute an improved state of affairs for all stakeholders, whose interests and perceptions often differ widely. Service users, carers, neighbours and local community interests, hospital managers, different professions with their distinct yet complementary knowledge bases, police authorities, politicians and academics all offer observations and insights. The territory is vigorously contested. In the midst of this melee the mental health professional is increasingly subject to more rigorous forms of bureaucratic surveillance, ever wary and arguably much less inclined toward therapeutic risk-taking.

Negotiating the care/control tension has become a central focus of work with those with serious mental illness and increased preoccupation with the management of risk means that training and professional updating in such areas has become a mandatory requirement for clinical professionals. Some have been able to avoid it or side-step it more easily than others (psychology professionals notably) whilst some others, who are immersed in it, may long to detach themselves from it. (Some psychiatrists in the UK currently long for this exemption). Such luxury is not afforded the case manager or care co-ordinator whose daily routines require constant negotiation of the tension. Pilgrim (1999) argues that both politicians and professionals show an unwillingness to acknowledge the control dimension of mental health services and that this constitutes both 'conceptual dishonesty' and contributes to the over-medicalisation of 'deviant conduct' in the sense that it contributes to the casting of much rule-violating conduct as 'illness behaviour requiring care'. The 'conceptual dishonesty' becomes all the more visible as the power of psychiatry becomes ever more transparent and subject to greater pressure for accountability, and where an increasingly explicit recognition exists that mental health services work sometimes in the interests of 3rd parties (relatives, the general public, the police, the criminal justice system and clinical professional interests).

The increasing pressure for public services to have their performance or 'success' exposed to evaluation at a number of levels is an additional dimension. The so called 'management of risk' is one major area where all the public services are increasingly subject to scrutiny and are held accountable and publicly vilified, if exposed when retrospectively deficits are discovered. Ironically as belief in the 'expertise' of professionals has undergone progressive erosion, the political expectations of 'professional expertise' in providing knowledge for risk management purposes has increased. In the UK recent trends in clinical governance linked to the need for organisational insurance against potential negligence claims highlight the necessity for robust risk management procedures as a vital concern of all mental health providers. In parts of the US this has gone to marked extremes such that the discharge of patients with particular risk histories from hospital inpatient settings without the advice and scrutiny of discharge plans by the hospital attorney would be unthinkable (Foster, 2001). Increasingly such developments condition the climate within which professionals in the US, UK and Australia work.

At the same time risk has increasingly become the most important criterion for eligibility or entitlement to services and thus the allocation of scarce resources. It follows that to be defined as 'low risk' is to be 'less eligible' for support. It is perhaps no accident that the rationing of entitlement in this way has occurred in the context of the implementation in all three societies of an explicitly neo-liberal agenda in relation to welfare policy, a retreat from the universalistic emphasis of the past. The fact that a preoccupation with the definition and management of risk also serves the purpose of defining and legitimating rationing has not gone unnoticed by some commentators. Indeed the political imperative of cost containment is cited as an overall context of mental health policy and reform by Shera, Healy, Aviram and Ramon (2002) in their four-nation comparison and also by Hollingsworth (1994) who observes that the decade of the 1980s saw an overall decline in funding for the care of the mentally ill in the US.

Rose (1998 and 2000) attempts a sociological unpicking of how the problematic of risk and its control has come to dominate the territory of contemporary psychiatric professionals. His argument is framed in terms of the re-casting of social problems in increasingly competitive liberal market economies as 'the problem of the excluded'. The changing roles of mental health professionals and their increasing designation as 'managers of risk' is seen as relating to much wider political and economic processes which bear on the sociology of governance. At the same time as these processes become more explicit and observable in all three societies there have emerged in parallel, and unacknowledged by Rose, new forces which seek to empower consumers of services, challenge stigma and discrimination and sustain agendas which are socially inclusive (HMSO, 2004). With the exception of the US Disability Discrimination legislation (Sayce, 2000) which does appear to have real legal teeth, such developments often fall short of legal entitlement with full redress for the disenfranchised but do represent powerful politically backed efforts to sustain a vision of services which empower, enable and reintegrate as well as 'control'. In all three societies the implementation of assertive community treatment has seen more intensive forms of support emerge, with a focus on holistic care and close attention to the everyday living support and skills. Attention to housing, income, education and training as well as community participation and varieties of supported employment is arguably leading to a more explicitly psychosocial focus. The evolution toward 24/7 services, meaningful alternatives to hospital admission and the adoption by psychiatrists of methods of working which reflect a 'recovery' as opposed to an 'illness' dominated model of mental health care are evidenced in a less substantial way with considerable variation within and between societies, however, the standard elements of provision do show some convergence, along with the rhetoric of policy and practice in all three societies. Despite this, the wider service contexts differ importantly in certain respects, with varying forms of legal regulation, compulsion and control over citizenship rights and connectedly over the treatment modalities which consumers may be able to access or find themselves compelled to accept.

The following case study/scenarios have been developed to illustrate some of the tensions and comparative differences. It is a fictitious case study though it will have resonance with the experience of most professionals working at the chalk face in community mental health service provision. The scenarios have been developed in partnership with colleagues in South Australia (Adelaide) and USA (New Hampshire) where legal devices for compulsory treatment in community settings have been commonly used for the last decade. Community Treatment Orders have been used in South Australia since 1993 and the Conditional Discharge legislation in New Hampshire since the mid 1990s. Both provide for quite explicit coercive powers. In all three scenarios the professionals involved are balancing a range of rights and responsibilities not just in relation to the various stakeholders but also in relation to their own organisational roles and liabilities. The matters at stake include invasion of privacy, detention and deprivation of liberty, the protection of other persons, the compulsory use of medication, physical restraint, the possibility of reprisal, the safety of housing tenure, the management of money, the control of future behaviour through engagement, negotiation and real or actual threat and access to community support in its various forms. Complex information sharing protocols exist which guide the actions of professionals in on the spot decisions about the sharing of normally confidential health care information with others who may have 'a need to know'. This activity is mandated by the 'duty of care' to the patient and to others. In all three societies the case manager/care co-ordinator is located precisely at this nexus of care and control.

Case Study

Peter has a diagnosis of bi-polar depression complicated by periods of alcohol and illicit drug (cannabis and amphetamine) usage, the onset of which is closely related to relapse. He has a history of hospital presentations at times of crisis, presenting mostly at the hospital Accident and Emergency department having been picked up by the police in public places in a distressed state complaining about voices in his head. Recently the police were called to his home following a dispute between Peter and his father which involved Peter threatening to use a knife. Peter refuses to allow access to mental health professionals when he is unwell, whether this is a nurse, social worker or community support worker, and although he has had periods of relative stability on medication in the past, he is currently refusing to take his medication and also refusing to attend psychiatric outpatient appointments. He believes that he is perfectly well, though neighbours and close family have witnessed recent ominous signs which have previously indicated a crisis is imminent and believe that he needs urgent help before he harms himself or someone else. Peter's mother, who lives close by, believes that he is not eating properly and that his flat is in a mess and bills remain unpaid. These are also warning signs evidenced in the past. His self-care has deteriorated and neighbours report that he is 'up all night' playing loud music and only leaving the house periodically for visits to the Off Licence. Yesterday, in the early hours of the morning, Peter fled from his flat to seek the assistance of a neighbour. He had, it would seem, left a pan on a lighted stove and it had burnt dry. Black smoke was seen billowing from his window. Neighbours called an ambulance and Peter was taken to hospital A&E department suffering from the effects of smoke inhalation. Following some three hours in A&E a junior doctor insisted that Peter be seen by the psychiatric liaison team. Not fully aware of what this implied, Peter agreed to be seen, but when a liaison nurse suggested that Peter he seen by a psychiatrist he promptly left the hospital.

UK Scenario

Though Peter may have committed an offence the police are reluctant to arrest him because he is known to have 'mental health problems' and the Crown Prosecution service, who make the final decisions about the viability of a prosecution, are unlikely to agree to proceed, claiming that such a prosecution might not be 'in the public interest'. The police also refuse to pick him up under the provisions of S136 of the Mental Health Act (1983) because when they last saw him he 'seemed fine' and on two previous occasions when S136 of the Act had been invoked, psychiatrists had refused to assess him because of high levels of intoxication. Though the Act permits such a detention for a period of up to 72 hours the police are very reluctant to hang around in a hospital A&E department for someone like Peter to become sufficiently sober to assess, the pressure of other police duties being too great.

Peter's mother, on the advice of her GP (who is also Peter's GP) rings the community mental health team and says that Peter needs to be in hospital but she does not want him to know that she has rung because of fear of reprisal. She is Peter's 'Nearest Relative' under the Mental Health Act, being the elder of his two parents. The CMHT duty worker liases with the GP who believes that an assessment for compulsory admission under the Mental Health Act is required but he himself is not willing to be involved because he has not seen Peter recently and because of 'pressure of time'. He also mentions that his involvement in such matters is not a mandatory requirement of his contract with the NHS so even if his involvement should be encouraged as 'best practice' he is not legally bound to attend.

The following day, after discussion with the duty psychiatrist, the duty ASW (Approved Social Worker) decides to convene an assessment under the Mental Health Act. Since the GP will not participate there is a need to locate a doctor approved under S12 of the Act to accompany the ASW and the duty psychiatrist. This takes some hours but eventually a doctor is located and the team convenes outside Peter's flat (with a discreet police presence) in the late afternoon. They arrive to find Peter returning from a shopping trip. He bluntly refuses to speak to the assessors, denies them access and slams the door shut.

The team decide that the ASW should seek a warrant (MH Act, 1983: S135 (1)) from the Magistrates court in order to gain access. The ASW achieves this the following morning, but not without difficulty as the Clerk to the Magistrates has recently been on some training in relation to the incorporation of European Human Rights legislation into UK law. He believes that Peter should possibly have been informed 'in writing' of the intention to seek a warrant. Clarification of this causes delay. In possession of the warrant the ASW convenes two further assessments on successive days. At the third attempt Peter is found at home and he is detained for treatment under S3 of the 1983 Act. Two medical recommendations deem Peter to have 'a mental disorder of a nature and degree' which warrants detention under the Act and that such a detention is necessary in the interests of his own health and safety and the safety of other persons. The ASW does not believe that his needs can be met by any viable alternative resource to that provided by an inpatient admission so she makes the application to the hospital managers for his admission. Peter is made subject to a treatment order, which can last up to 12 months if the conditions for detention persist. He is conveyed to hospital in the rear of a police car accompanied by two police officers as the ambulance service, on hearing of recent events, refuse to transport him because of possible risks to themselves. Peter's community RMO remains responsible for his inpatient care throughout the duration of his stay.

Some three weeks into his treatment, having become well enough to access the advice of an advocate and appreciate fully his rights to challenge his detention

Peter decides to make an application to a Mental Health Tribunal with full legal representation, however, he withdraws his application after attending a ward round where it is agreed that he is well enough for his section to be lifted. This happens the day before his Tribunal hearing is due.

Following four weeks of inpatient treatment Peter is ready for discharge, his mood having stabilised and his agreement secured to a detailed care plan entailing medication management and monitoring, housing support, referral to a day programme to address his substance misuse and agreement to work on relapse prevention strategies with appropriate crisis and contingency plans. Such planning is a requirement of discharge under S117 of the Act and appropriate to Peter's status as an enhanced user of services under the Care Programme Approach (CPA). His mother is invited to attend the discharge meeting but declines to do so. His care co-ordinator, a community psychiatric nurse, is responsible for networking with relevant providers and ensuring the care plan is delivered and well communicated to relevant parties. Team members who know Peter feel that his 'agreement' to this plan will be rapidly tested and there is some debate in the team about the possible use of S25a of the 1983 Act (Supervised Discharge), but the team psychiatrist (as Responsible Medical Officer) is reluctant to agree to this believing that it might 'damage therapeutic relationships' and that it only provides for 'a power to convey' (to a place of treatment) and that Peter is 'intelligent enough to know this'.

Peter is discharged with his S117 package of support in place. He attends one follow-up outpatient appointment and refuses to agree to his care co-ordinators suggestion that the local authority become appointee for his social security benefits. After a month he disengages from contact with his care co-ordinator and ceases to attend the drug and alcohol day services programme. An onward referral is made to the Assertive outreach team to attempt to engage him further.

Peter resumes his claim for Disability Living allowance which had been temporarily suspended during his inpatient admission. CMHT (community mental health team) workers reluctantly acknowledge the high probability that much of this money will continue to be spent in a manner harmful to Peter's health. The capped caseloads of the AOT, (assertive outreach team) a greater likelihood of expertise in supporting the dually diagnosed, and a team determination to engage with Peter 'on his own terms' may increase the chances of therapeutic success in the future but the current legal framework will not prevent a reoccurrence of the events described above.

USA: The New Hampshire Scenario

Peter's mother and father contact the Community Mental Health Centre on the advice of the Chief of Police who sits on the team's Board of Governors. On hearing of the parents concerns and after speaking with local police officers the assessment team agree to act as petitioners to pursue an Involuntary Emergency Admission. For this to be actioned a full medical examination is required. Peter refuses to participate in the medical examination and the team files a 'Prayer and Complaint' with the local justice after which the local police pick Peter up from his flat and transport him to the local Community Mental Health Centre or local hospital emergency room. In transit Peter may be handcuffed if he is agitated or threatens to harm police officers. Peter is examined by a doctor and subsequently admitted to the New Hampshire Hospital. The hospital has a statutory responsibility to provide a bed and has been fully briefed by the community team. With legal representation Peter attends a 'Probable Cause' Hearing in the hospital district courtroom within 72 hours.

'Probable Cause' is found and Peter's detention continues for a maximum of 10 days from the initial admission. Peter is distressed and angry, refusing all offers of medication and at one point he is deemed as 'needing seclusion and restraint'. The hospital file a petition for a Non-Emergency Involuntary Admission and some 12 days later a full Probate Court hearing takes place at which Peter receives full legal representation and an independent medical examiner provides evidence for the court's deliberations. At the same time the hospital presents evidence to the court in relation to Peter's 'lack of capacity' over health care decisions and financial matters. He has many unpaid bills and there is evidence of a history of misuse of his social security money on drugs and alcohol to the extent that his mental and physical health are prejudiced.

The Court finds that the conditions are met for a Non-Emergency Involuntary admission and proceeds with the appointment of a Guardian from the approved list. Medication cannot be forcefully administered against the patient's expressed wishes until this is done. Peter wishes his mother to be appointed as Guardian but she declines. Had she agreed the Court might still have overruled this as being in neither the patient nor his mother's 'best interests'. Since Peter's 'Commitment' is to the community mental health system and not to the hospital as such, he may be conditionally discharged to the care of his local community team on terms negotiated by himself, the state Hospital and the community team. This could mean that his period of compulsory hospitalisation could be quite brief though technically he would remain, subsequently, subject to the compulsory powers associated with conditional discharge. He could be asked to take his medication 'as required', allow access to team clinicians and support workers and also to start to address his drug and alcohol usage by attendance at designated rehabilitation programmes, either on a day basis or possibly, for a period, residentially. On discharge should Peter fail to comply with crucial elements of the care plan, he runs the risk of his case manager seeking the revocation of his discharge. This is a 'stepped' process with procedures on a continuum from witnessed oral warnings to full statutory revocation and re-committal readmission to the state hospital.

With the consent of his Guardian and on the recommendation of the responsible psychiatrist, Peter's benefits may be administered by the Mental Health Centre, with it becoming the payee for his social security. Domestic bills would be paid on his behalf and he would be left with a small weekly allowance to meet personal needs. A 'representative payee' within the CMHT performs these functions so that they are not added to the responsibilities of case managers or care-co-ordinators.

Peter is likely to become a client of a Continuous Treatment Team operating on assertive outreach principles and supported by Housing Outreach workers and vocational, rehabilitation specialists. Strenuous efforts will be made to support him into sheltered and/or paid work as part of the rehabilitation/community treatment process. Case managers will be dually trained in mental health and drug/alcohol treatment interventions and motivational interviewing techniques and probably benefit from the skill and knowledge of a team psychiatrist who accept works with the dually diagnosed as part of his/her territory.

This scenario demonstrates a subtle balance of coercion and negotiated consent in the treatment process, reflecting a preoccupation with the management of risk through an explicitly judicial process with the potential to remove a range of civil rights for those who either refuse or are unable to comply with the specific behavioural expectations identified in the conditional discharge.

The South Australia Scenario

Peter's mother contacts the Assessment and Crisis Intervention Service (ACIS) of the Mental Health Service (a 24-hour telephone service and 16 hours per day 7 days per week mobile service) on the advice of the local police. The police will not take any action over the knife incident unless Peter's father wishes to press charges. The police also believe there is insufficient evidence to take Peter for a mental health assessment under Section 23 of the South Australian Mental Health Act 1993, as he was calm and co-operative with them.

The ACIS telephone triage worker takes the history from Peter's mother and decides that an assessment is warranted and arranges this for the following morning. The ACIS worker, as part of the triage, does a telephone risk assessment and determines that the risk category is high and that police will need to be present during the assessment. As Peter's mother does not wish to be the identified referrer the ACIS worker contacts the police who agree to be the referring agent and also agree to attend with the ACIS staff the next day. The ACIS team will consist of a psychiatric registrar and mental health nurse. The worker also contacts Peter's GP to inform him of the referral and to glean any background information the GP may be able to provide. The case is discussed at the ACIS clinical meeting the following morning and the plan remains the same.

On arrival at Peter's home the ACIS staff identify themselves but he refuses to open the door. The ACIS staff persist, with eventually the police convinces Peter to open the door. An assessment is conducted and it is clear that Peter is delusional and quite unwell. The registrar offers Peter voluntary community treatment but he refuses and is unwilling to engage further. Given the events leading up-to the referral and his current mental state the registrar decides to detain Peter under the Mental Health Act (1993) on a Form 1 (an order for immediate admission to an approved treatment centre). The registrar also completes a Form 15 (a conveyance authority) and an ambulance is called and Peter is conveyed to the approved treatment centre (hospital) for the area in which he lives. The police follow behind. The ambulance takes Peter to the emergency department for a thorough physical examination prior to admission to the nominated acute psychiatric ward. On arrival at the ward the ward's admitting psychiatric registrar formally admits Peter to the ward. Peter's family and GP are informed of his admission.

The following morning Peter is reviewed by one of the ward's consultant psychiatrists. This is a mandatory process to determine whether Peter can be discharged to community care, including continuing admission through the Hospital at Home programme, or that the detention order remains and is extended or the order is revoked and Peter remains as a voluntary in-patient. The psychiatrist believes that Peter requires a further period of detention for further assessment and treatment as Peter is unwilling to engage in voluntary treatment. The order is extended for a further 72 hours on a Form 2, the maximum allowable at this time. During the next 3 days continuing assessment, treatment and observation is conducted. Nearing the end of the 72 hours Peter is again formally assessed by the psychiatrist to decide again if he can be discharged, requires further detention, can be transferred to the Hospital at Home Programme or remain as a voluntary patient. However, the psychiatrist extends the order on a Form 3 for a further 21 days, which is the maximum allowable at this time. Peter is informed that this order can be revoked at any time during the 21 days and also of his right of appeal.

The treating team are planning for discharge in about seven days. The team are not confident that Peter will voluntarily engage with community follow-up and given the lead-up to this admission, apply to the Guardianship Board of South Australia for a Treatment Order, to provide treatment against Peter's wishes if he does not voluntarily engage, and also an Administration Order, to allow the Public Trustee of South Australia to manage Peter's finances so that his bills are paid for him reducing the risk of homelessness. (The Board only has jurisdiction in South Australia.)

The Board hearing is set for about four weeks time. The ward treating team are wanting to discharge Peter before this and as part of the discharge planning refer Peter to the Mobile Assertive Care Service (MACS), a seven day per week assertive follow-up service) and one of the MACS workers attends the ward to meet Peter. They envisage Peter will require depot medication and commence this on the ward while he is still detained. After ten days the psychiatrist revokes Peter's detention and discharges him from hospital to the MACS. The team takes Peter on immediately.

The inpatient registrar who was managing Peter on the ward and the ward social worker attend the Guardianship Board hearing. As is his right and choice, Peter attends with legal representation from Legal Aid, a government funded legal service for people who cannot afford a lawyer. (The Guardianship Board hearing is not a court of law and is not part of the judicial system). The application is successful on both counts and the Orders are granted for 12 months (the maximum allowable), which means Peter must adhere to the treatment prescribed by the treating doctor. Failure to do so could mean police notification and conveyance by police to the clinic, and if necessary the authority can be given for Peter to be readmitted to hospital if he fails to comply and his mental state deteriorates.

However, Peter understands these conditions and complies. The MACS appoints a care co-ordinator to oversee his general community care plan and sees

Peter initially four times per week. Peter also has appointments either at home or the clinic with the team's psychiatrist fortnightly. The care co-ordinator has regular contact with Peter's Public Trustee Officer to ensure Peter's finances are structured in a manner that allows for bills to be paid and that he has a weekly allowance paid into his bank account for personal use. His parents and GP are kept informed of progress.

It is anticipated Peter will be with the MACS for about 6–9 months before being transferred to another CMHT within the service, where he will receive a less intensive/assertive service. Over time with the MACS Peter will be re-engaged with his GP and the frequency of contact with his worker and doctor appointments will be reduced as his mental state and level of functioning improves. Every effort will be made to keep Peter in independent living. This may include applying for funds to provide a housing support worker to come in a few hours per week to help Peter keep his house clean and tidy and also to assist with shopping. If independent living is not sustainable then referral to a community Supported Residential Facility may be needed.

The CMHT can reapply at the end of the 12 months to the Board for continuation of the Treatment Order or allow it to lapse. This will depend on what the clinical picture looks like for Peter at this time and how successfully he has engaged in treatment.

Comment

Case study/scenarios of this kind clearly have limitations in that they can really only serve to highlight the legal and service frameworks within which treatment is provided and therapeutic relationships forged. They pinpoint issues that need exploration in much more depth and with greater rigour. Currently in the UK with a revised Mental Health Bill once more on the agenda the spectre of enhanced controls in community settings is raised again with service users and key professionals concerned about the possible impacts.

In many States of the US there exist forms of legal regulation which provide for significant powers of compulsion outside hospital settings, together with robust forms of Guardianship which divest a service user of a range of rights which are subsequently vested in another person though such processes are firmly subject to judicial processes and regular review. Such rights include those in relation to choices about residence, housing, healthcare, management of finances and even relationship choices.

Despite the rhetoric of a US system driven by evidence as to 'cost effectiveness', 'efficiency' and 'measurable outcomes', there is surprisingly little conclusive data in relation to what must be considered a key element of the 'containment and control' agenda, namely compulsory commitment to community treatment (30 states have provision for this though only 12 use it commonly) or the form of conditional discharge from hospital subject to adherence to release conditions (40 states have provision for this). Leading clinicians are themselves cautious in the claims they make about the efficacy of such powers. Drake and Mueser and Noordsy (1988) note that:

> Coercive interventions such as involuntary hospitalisation, guardianship or commitment to community treatment are sometimes necessary to stabilise the dangerously ill dually diagnosed patient. It is important to recognise that the prevention of harm and compulsory compliance that involuntary measures may provide do not constitute treatment and that such controls may hold a patient static at best (see also Mueser, 1997).

In New Hampshire the robust Conditional Discharge legislation was passed through the state legislature with strong political pressure from relatives and carers organisations (notably the National Alliance for the Mentally Ill) and became law against the expressed wishes of users themselves. South Australia likewise, as the case study indicates, has compulsory community treatment as a central plank of its legal regulation over the lives of the seriously mentally ill together with significant powers attaching to the office of the Public Trustee to manage the finances of a service user such as Peter. Australia has evolved and implemented forms of coercive legal regulation which afford considerably greater scope for the power to enforce treatment in community settings than exist in either the UK or the US. The use of CTOs (Community Treatment Orders) is widespread in both South Australia and the neighbouring states of New South Wales and Victoria (see Healy and Brophy, 2000) without the kind of exacting judicially regulated oversight characteristic of comparable legislation in the USA. This appears to have happened without concerted public outcry and concern but is clearly deeply resented by many users of mental health services. Brophy, Campbell and Healy (2003) note how the existing literature provides a wide range of views on the potential benefits and drawbacks of compulsion in community settings, embracing such concerns as efficacy, social justice and human rights and the serious ethical dilemmas faced by professionals in employing such methods of control. Significant claims have been made in relation to reduced length of hospitalisation (Jarorowski and Guneva, 2002), preventing disengagement following discharge (Lee, 1993), their evolution as part of a wider risk management endeavour (Rose, 1998) and even claims that the use of such powers facilitates greater 'insight' in service users (McIvor, 1998). Brophy *et al.*, also, however, cite a range of evidence which might encourage a more sceptical attitude, including that by Preston (2002) in which a survey of 456 patients in Western Australia suggested that there was some evidence that CTOs led to a reduction in the use of wider mental health services and that they may not be more effective in achieving better health outcomes than assertive outreach.

In all three societies we see stark reminders of the power of psychiatry to treat against the expressed wishes of the patient and to define the limits within which individuals with an identified mental illness might have their basic rights as citizens eroded in various respects, whether the rights are withdrawn in explicitly legally regulated ways or whether they are implicitly invaded by various forms of discretionary professional power, the use of which may serve to achieve behavioural compliance which might not otherwise be forthcoming. This is a unique situation in law and medicine and the case manager's location in this delicate and complex nexus puts him or her in a position which other professionals rarely savour.

There is perhaps some irony in the observation that the growth of viable community-based treatment alternatives which bring with them the potential for a more explicitly psychosocial model of intervention and governance would appear to be accompanied in the UK, Australia and the US by a widening of the scope for compulsion in non-institutional settings. Alongside the increasingly visible rhetoric of social inclusion, citizenship rights and wider scope for user and carer involvement and the embedding of consumer feedback in audit and practice governance systems, there coexists an equally visible agenda of risk management whose imperatives may signal very different messages. As the citizenship agenda seeks to protect rights and sustain a more empowering and integrating vision of entitlement to services with more flexible service delivery, greater accessibility, accountability and more respect for autonomy and self-determination one might hope that the reasons for people similar to Peter (the subject of our case study) coming to mistrust and fear statutory services may undergo some erosion. Recently a study by Watts and Priebe (2002) has sought to uncover some of the mechanisms which lead to 'disengagement', claiming that it is as much a historical and cultural phenomenon as it is a product of 'lack of insight'. In this study service users repeatedly reported experience of rejection of early help-seeking behaviour and all had been subject to coercive interventions which they had experienced as an attack on identity. Such research might suggest that previous experience of rejection and/or the use of compulsory powers may serve to sustain a view of services as both disinterested and coercive so that disengagement and the experience of coercion may often be causally linked.

It is hardly surprising then that the care/control tension remains so central to the ethics of community mental health and is likely to remain so for the foreseeable future. As Rose (1999: 261-262) comments:

> Psychiatry has long been as much an administrative as a clinical science. One only has to recall its relation to concerns about degeneration in the late nineteenth century, in eugenics strategies over the first half of the twentieth century, in programmes of mental hygiene in the 1930s and in plans for a comprehensive preventive health service in the 1950s and 60s under the sign of community psychiatry. The demand that psychiatry should be concerned with the assessment and administration of risky individuals rather than with diagnosis treatment and cure, does not mark a new moment in its political vocation. Nonetheless its role is revised in the new configuration of control. What is called for is the management of a permanently risky minority on the territory of the community.

Notes

Thanks to the following colleagues for assistance with this Chapter: Greg Calder (Western Community Mental Health Services, Adelaide, South Australia); David Pelletier (West Central Services, Psychiatric Research Centre, Lebanon, New

Hampshire); Lisa Brophy (NorthWestern Mental Health, Melbourne, Victoria, Australia).

References

Brophy, L., Campbell, J. and Healy, B. (2003), 'Dilemmas in the case manager's role: implementing involuntary treatment in the community', *Psychiatry, Psychology and the Law*. Vol. 10(1), 154-164.

Drake. B., Mueser. K. and Noordsy. D. (1988), 'Integrated mental health and substance abuse treatment for severe psychiatric disorders'. *Journal of Practical Psychiatry and Behavioural Health*.

Foster, N. (2001), 'Involuntary outpatient commitment: Managing mental health risks the New Hampshire way'. *Journal of Mental Health and Learning Disabilities Care*. Vol. 4, Issue 11.

Healy, B. and Brophy, L. (2001), 'Law psychiatry and social work'. In Swain, P. (ed.) *In the Shadow of the Law*. Sydney. The Federation Press.

HMSO (2004), *Mental Health and Social Exclusion*.

HMSO (2004), *Action on Mental Health: A Guide to Promoting Social Exclusion*.

Hollingsworth, E. (1994), 'Falling through the cracks: Care of the chronically mentally ill in the US'. In Hollingsworth, J. and Hollingsworth, E. *Care of the Chronically and Severely Ill*, Walter Gruyter Inc. New York.

Jaworowski, S. and Guneva, R. (2002), 'Decision-making in Community Treatment Orders: A comparison of clinicians and Mental Health Review Board members'. *Australian Psychiatry*, 10(1).

Lee, J. (1993), Community Treatment Orders: The Victorian experience. *Health Issues*.

McIvor, R. (1998), 'The community treatment order: Clinical and ethical issues'. *Australian and New Zealand Journal of Psychiatry*. 32, 223-228.

Mueser, K. *et al.* (1997), 'Treatment outcomes for seriously mentally ill patients on conditional discharge to community treatment'. *Journal of Nervous and Mental Disease*. 185, 409-411.

Pilgrim, D. (1999), 'Care, control and evidence in British mental health policy: The context for crisis services'. In Tomlinson, D. and Allen, K. (eds), *Crisis services and hospital crises: Mental health at the turning point*. Aldershot, Ashgate.

Preston, N.J., Kisely, S. and Xiao, J. (2002), 'Assessing the outcome of compulsory psychiatric treatment in the community: Epidemiological study in Western Australia'. *British Medical Journal*, Vol. 324, 1244-1249.

Rose, N. (1998), 'Governing risky individuals: The role of psychiatry in new regimes of control'. *Psychiatry, Psychology and the Law*. 5(2), 177-195.

Rose, N. (2000), *Powers of Freedom: Reframing Political Thought*. Cambridge, Cambridge University Press.

Sayce, L. (2000), *From Psychiatric Patient to Citizen: Overcoming Discrimination and Social Exclusion*. Basingstoke, Macmillan.

Shera, W., Healy, B., Aviram, U. and Ramon, S. (2002), 'Mental Health Policy and Practice: a multi-country comparison'. *Journal of Health and Mental Health Social Work*. 35, 1-2, 547-575.

Watt, J. and Priebe, S. (2002), 'A phenomenological account of users experiences of assertive community treatment'. *Bioethics* 16/5, 439-54.

Chapter 3

Contextualised Social Policy:
An Australian Perspective

Bill Healy and Noel Renouf

Introduction

Mental health policy and programmes in Australia have over the past 50 years undergone an enormous range of changes. In essence they have moved from a system dominated by large congregate care institutions to one defined as being a set of essential community-based programmes. This pattern of change is typically presented as being a linear, progressive triumph of advances in biological-medical understandings of and responses to major mental illness and the result of caring and committed governments. It is our contention that the story is much more complex, messy and non-linear and the result of change happening in often-turbulent environments. More often 'progress' has been disorganised, recursive and the product of enduring tensions between the competing interests (care, control, protection and treatment) and the underpinning ideological and theoretical paradigms (psychological, social, legal and biological-medical) of understanding and action in response to the social problem of mental health and mental illness (Bainbridge, 1999; Healy, 2002; Meadows and Singh, 2001).

At some points in our local history these different interests and approaches to policy and service arrangements seem to have been in relative harmony. For instance some 50 years ago following very public exposure of appalling physical conditions and the almost total lack of treatment for patients in the mental hospitals in one Australian state, Victoria, a major reform was undertaken under the banner of social psychiatry (Dax, 1992). The resultant changes preceded the introduction of the modern psychotropic medications, were primarily focussed on improvements to the conditions of the old institutions so that patients had better accommodation, food, more privileges, less restrictions on their movements and significantly more connection with the wider community (Dax, 1961). At the same time the reforms also sensibly sought to greatly improve the range and quality of staff, especially medical and nursing, and placed faith in system improvement due to a major upgrade of education, training and research.

At other times the nature and direction of change has been more the result of, or has led to, the exacerbation of the tensions between the identified range of interests and approaches to policy and programme development in the mental health field. Current conditions seem to represent a pattern of 'progress' which is underpinned by a number of, more or less explicit, conflictual sets of circumstances on the one hand, around balancing out the competing interests of care and community concern, and on the other hand around the competing definitions of what constitutes the system's preferred mode of intervention with identified consumers (the preferred – but contentious – Australian term for service users). In order to better understand this story it is necessary to go back to the first National Mental Health Plan, and its component parts, namely the Strategy and the Policy of 1992 (Australian Health Ministers, 1992). Until that time mental health services were virtually the sole responsibility of the Australian States and Territories with the Commonwealth Government playing only a minor role.

This chapter focuses on the policy for services for adults between 18 and 65 which is probably the area that is most contested in Australia in relation to the competing paradigms of medical-biological approaches and psychosocial approaches.

Current Policy Directions

A mix of aims, interests and motives drove the first National Mental Health Plan of 1992. There was, for instance, considerable recognition that services were poorly funded, anachronistic in their reliance on institutional care and offering a type and quality of service, which was significantly poorer than was the case in general health. At the same time the process of deinstitutionalisation, which had been a reality, albeit a slow moving one, for some years, was accelerating to such an extent that the imminent closures of institutions required additional resources to carry the massive shifts of the locus and focus to community settings. This policy outcome has been frequently represented as an agreement between the Commonwealth and the States that would precipitate a more rapid modernisation of services in return for increased funding from the Centre (Meadows and Singh, 2001).

Thus the first national policy gave a central role to two key concepts, mainstreaming and integration (Healy and Varney, 1995). The former was the policy aim of moving mental health services from their isolated and separatist existence in the old institutions into the context of health policy and service provision. The latter was a recognition that services had to be vertically integrated across a range of mental health programmes which were to be based in both general hospital and community settings and which related to a notion of essential continuity of care. Thus improved inpatient services are proposed to be based in general hospitals and the range of other related services to be delivered primarily through redeployed public sector organisations but now with the emergence of some acknowledgement of other stakeholders, namely, consumers, the NGO or non-government sector and private agencies. In short the primary focus of this first national policy was upon building a better structure of services, which met the needs of consumers and the wider community in a post-institutional world (Whiteford *et al.*, 2002).

The implementation was overtaken by a variety of contextual issues. Most importantly it coincided with massive neo-liberal reform of government, which led to extensive restructures of public organisations, significant reduction in budget commitments, a rush to contract out services and resultant major changes in work practices. In these contexts, the psychosocial interests embedded in the National Plan became diminished and at the same time, the seemingly more efficient medical interventions became more dominant.

The second National Plan of 1998 identified further priority areas for reform and in particular identified promotion and prevention; the building of better partnerships across related service areas; and increased quality and effectiveness of services. To some extent this iteration of national policy made the psychosocial interests more explicit. The choice of these goals reflected a combination of the identification of continuing problems of quality; the WHO agenda that has focussed on the notion of burden of disease; and the recognition that outcomes ultimately relate far more to quality of life than they do to levels of symptomatology (Australian Health Ministers, 1998). The new emphasis on early intervention and primary prevention draws on a public health, population based approach that means that the second National Mental Health Strategy provides:

> ... a broader focus, with stronger emphasis on population health issues and interventions. To a large extent this is both inevitable and desirable. Stemming from the Strategy's initial concern with the long-term mentally ill, it is necessary that any modern nation widen its concern to mental health issues in the community and the social, political and economic forces that produce mental health disorder. The emphasis on a 'whole of community' approach to building resilience and reducing future community morbidity is also consistent with World Bank projections of an increase over the next 20 years in the burden associated with mental illnesses (Commonwealth Department of Health and Aged Care, 2000: 14).

A further aspect of this recognition of the community care base to the new mental health services is the priority given to the primary care sector. Most often this means that the mental health consumer's first line of referral and subsequent continuing care is with their local general practitioner. In recognition of this renewed emphasis on the role of primary care providers the policy also encourages the creation of specialist mental health teams to support the sector. In the authors' State, Victoria, these are known as the 'Primary Mental Health Team' and are now operating across the whole system. Once again there is both recognition of, and a tension between, the competing paradigms as well as fiscal issues at work. That is in relation to costs it is clear that there is embedded in the policy a reliance on eventual savings, in terms of an anticipated reduction in the degree of the burden of disease costs, as the result of supporting general practitioners and community health agencies to provide services to people with high prevalence disorders as well as to those suffering from low prevalence disorders. Generally the favoured model underlying interventions is a mix of medication and psychological measures, most notably cognitive behavioural therapy, but with little emphasis on any significant social interventions, despite local evidence of the social and psychological costs of mental ill health and the importance of related psychosocial interventions (Jablensky *et al.*, 1999; Hunter and Tsey, 2003).

For those suffering from low prevalence disorders there are some limited opportunities to access a variety of non-government mental health psychosocial rehabilitation programmes as well as a variety of mainstream health and welfare agencies which more or less follow a whole of life orientation to care and treatment. Whilst these have increased in range and number over recent years, not least because of the contracting out of services that are a feature of neo-liberal reform of government, they still remain a small part of the overall mental health system (Commonwealth Department of Health and Aged Care, 2000).

New and Enduring Challenges

A welcome consequence of the national policy initiatives of the past decade has been a very large increase in the emphases, both policy and budgetary, given to the demographic, ethnic and cultural diversity of Australia. It is now common to read in policy documents and in academic papers (Collinson and Copolov, 2004) references to the special needs of people in relation to their social status and related needs. A recent supplement of Australasian Psychiatry (Hunter and Walter, 2003) contains a selection of papers, presented at a National Conference of the Social and Cultural Section of the Australian and New Zealand College of Psychiatry, on indigenous populations, consumers, refugees and detained populations and rural and remote populations. A recent review of desirable research opportunities in mental health research in Australia (Collinson and Copolov, 2004) highlights the distinctive population mix of Australian society which includes a significant indigenous population, an ageing 'old' European population, a continuing immigrant intake which more recently has had additional numbers of people from Asia and a refugee intake policy which more recently has seen arrivals from the Middle East, Africa and Asia. This latter group, many of whom are detainees, have become a focus of concern, for diametrically different reasons, for many mental health professionals and the Commonwealth government. In this instance the conflict at a policy and programme level is between the concerns of the professionals for the profound psychological, physical and social impacts of detention upon detainees and the contradictory way in which government applies different standards of care and protection to those which exist in the wider community (Dudley, 2003; Rees, 2003).

A further example of the intersection of political and managerial imperatives with a range of ideological approaches to mental health matters can be seen in the somewhat ambivalent practices in relation to consumer rights. It was not until 1975, and as late as the mid 1980s in some jurisdictions, that a mental health act in Australia made mention of patient's rights and began to remove the limitations on patients that resulted from involuntary status including the right to manage their own finances and property, enter into contracts and to vote, all in the context of no judicial or administrative legal review (Healy and Brophy, 2002). Since 1992 there has been a model of rights policy and practice through the UN Principles for the Protection of the Rights of the Mentally Ill (Zifcak, 1996) and as a part of

Australia's treaty obligations is required to be incorporated into each State's Mental Health legislation.

Despite this progress the Australian Human Rights and Equal Opportunity Commission Inquiry into the Rights of the Mentally Ill (HREOC, 1993) delivered a damning indictment of what it judged to be the low level of not only adherence to rights but also both the quality and quantity of services and the almost total lack of any recognition in legislation or policy of the right to treatment. The impact of this and a later HREOC Report are difficult to gauge although the Chairman of the Inquiry, Brian Burdekin, was reported some years later in *The Age* newspaper as stating that little has changed in the intervening years:

> Unfortunately since that report ... a lot of things may have changed but the sad reality ... (is) hundreds of thousands of Australians affected by mental illness are still being relegated to a role of third-class citizens (Burdekin, 2001).

Whilst the closures of the old institutions and the development of extensive community based services have been widely welcomed they also have raised the level of anxiety within government about risk and even the dangers, principally political, that adhere to the perception of risk within the community. One result has been that all States in Australia have now legislated to enable compulsory treatment in the community and have dramatically increased the numbers on such orders at a rate commensurate with the rate of closures of the large institutions (Healy and Brophy, 2002). This emphasis on risk management has greatly increased the pressure for case managers and others to give priority to a focus on risk assessment and as a consequence has reduced much of the concern of service provision to monitoring medication compliance.

Tensions in Implementation

Under Australia's Federal system of government, the implementation of National Mental Health Policy has occurred unevenly in the various States and Territories, and – in some cases – unevenly within those States. For example, total expenditure on specialised mental health services varies substantially from $96 per head of population per year in Western Australia, to $67 per head in the Australian Capital Territory, and there has been significant variation in the manner and degree of implementation of community-based services (Commonwealth Department of Health and Ageing, 2002).

Case Management

Perhaps the clearest policy directions have been those of the Victorian Government, which introduced a 'Framework' for service delivery in 1994 that divided the state into defined service areas of approximately 200,000 people, and required that each service area provide the following range of mental health services (Psychiatric Services Division, Victorian Government Department of Health and Community Services, 1994):

- A mobile crisis assessment and community treatment team
- An acute inpatient ward in a general hospital, with access to a small number of secure extended care beds
- Specialist community mental health teams working through a case management model
- Mobile support and treatment teams for long-term intensive case management.

In addition, a range of regional or statewide services was established for groups such as people with co-occurring disorders, personality disorders, forensic clients, people from cultural and linguistically diverse backgrounds, and many others. Consistent with the thrust of prevailing neo-liberal reforms, services were funded through a purchaser-provider model that allowed the State considerable regulatory authority while shifting much of the responsibility for risk to other health care providers such as public hospitals and non-Government organisations.

Nevertheless, there has been a substantial achievement in moving from a hospital/institution based service system to one with much more emphasis on community-based services – primary care, specialist, and disability support, the latter being provided through non-government organisations. Specialist services in particular were significantly redeveloped in the First National Mental Health Plan to sharpen the focus on particular types of mental health problem (in most areas, so-called 'serious mental illness' – psychosis, major depression, certain forms of personality disorder) and to regulate the form of service provided. Of course, services differ in their level of intensity but, in general, the glue that holds together the speciality community mental health system in Australia is case management.

In the Victorian case, it is a requirement that every client of the specialist public mental health system have a case manager, with defined responsibilities. When the system was introduced in 1994, there was an extensive statewide training programme designed to build the capacity of the multidisciplinary workforce (many of whom had extensive experience in mental hospitals) in a model of clinical case management that emphasised the strengths of consumers, the importance of the helping relationship, and the collaborative achievement of goals documented in individual service plans that were comprehensive and included: emotional and mental wellbeing; dealing with stress; personal response to illness; personal safety and the safety of others; friendships/social relationships; work leisure and education; daily living skills; family's response to relative's illness; income; physical health; housing; and rights and advocacy (Victorian Government Department of Human Services, 1998). Clearly, such a model provides the opportunity to work with consumers to meet many of the wide range of needs that had been managed so minimally in the old institutional system.

At the same time, there was a clear imperative to establish case management as a mechanism for ensuring accountability for the risks associated with community mental health care – the risks of absent or inadequate treatment, and the risks of not meeting the competing needs and demands of service users, their families and people in their neighbourhoods. Case management was generally to be an individual responsibility: at least now, the responsibility would always be clear. The consequences on the service system have been considerable. Thus, for example, the working day in a busy Australian community mental health centre might begin with reports from the overnight crisis services – reports that threaten to bring unwelcome news of disturbance for each case manager. As the responsibilities of the community mental health service system have increased in the wake of de-institutionalisation – higher caseloads, less access to acute psychiatric hospital beds, increasingly well articulated demands from consumers, their families and the community, and a government sensitive to risk, there has been a strong, sometimes overwhelming tendency to retreat to a narrow definition of 'core business' – case-managing the illness, by means of the monitoring of symptoms and medication, rather than working collaboratively with the person. In any event, resources have not always kept pace with demand, and caseloads in some services have risen to the point that it is not possible for case managers to work with all consumers in the way that they would wish (Auditor General Victoria, 2002), especially in the context of a managerial culture that has not always fostered a supportive working environment. Thus, in various ways, each team and each case manager holds the tension of the contradiction between the emancipatory possibilities of clinical case management and the imperative of surveillance of risk. It is this tension that each referring agency, each consumer and each family meets in some form when they enter into a relationship with the community mental health service system as it has been designed. As a result this preoccupation with risk pervades the culture of everyday mental health work and results in conflict between the caring and controlling functions, inherent in policy, being enacted routinely at the site of the service provision with resulting distortion of the relationship between worker and consumer.

Consequences of the Mainstreaming Project

The stated aims of including the mental health services within the mainstream medical treatment system have been to reduce stigma and to improve standards. There is indeed modest evidence that standards have improved (Commonwealth Department of Health and Ageing, 2002), although the evidence that stigma has been reduced is equivocal at best (Carr and Halpin, 2002). Nor has mental health achieved parity in the funding terms, but rather its share of the health budget appears to have remained static. While mental health spending has been increasing in Australia, it accounts for approximately 7 per cent of the health budget while mental illness accounts for about 13 per cent of the total burden of disease and nearly 30 per cent of the non-fatal disease burden in Australia (Groom and Hickie, 2003).

The location of psychiatry, as a relatively low-status medical speciality, more firmly within the medical service system may have tended to push mental health services further away from an engagement with the social context and social consequences of mental health problems, and further towards the scientific and technical project of diagnosis, and medical and/or behavioural treatment based on 'evidence'. The dominant research paradigm is both a cause and a consequence of this focus, with an overwhelming concentration on pharmaceutical and other biological domains in the pursuit of knowledge about mental health. One consequence of mainstreaming is to buttress the power and influence of psychiatry, while making it more difficult to advance some of the public health policy agenda. In most parts of Australia, responsibility for mental health services sits with the larger hospital-based health services rather than with the smaller locally based community health system, which has stronger links with communities and local and natural support systems.

The system of universal health insurance, introduced in Australia in 1974 supported a flourishing, but poorly distributed and poorly regulated, system of private for-profit mental health services, that has to some extent served to complement the public system by providing specialist services for people who were excluded from public services with their resource constraints and narrowed focus. The more recent policy shift towards primary mental health has been clearly aimed at increasing the capacity of general practice doctors, with comparatively trivial attention being paid to non-medical community health services and even less to social care.

Improving outcomes for people with mental health problems typically involves the capacity to work creatively with them on housing, relationship, employment, spiritual and psychological issues as well as providing treatment for mental illness. Hence, services need to be set up in a way that values partnership as the fundamental basis of work with consumers, their families and communities, and emphasises work across sectors – incorporating expertise in dealing with alcohol and drug issues, housing, child welfare, income security, vocational support and so on. In each of these fields – constructed as they are by the logic of service systems as much as the logic of consumers' needs – there is a body of knowledge and practice expertise. The challenge for service design is to ensure that consumers have access to all of them together; for the service system, this means a capacity for effective cross-sector work. In the current Australian context this has proved to be particularly difficult to achieve (National Mental Health Strategy Evaluation Steering Committee for the Australian Health Ministers Advisory Council, 1997: 19-20), with the mental health system being drawn to a tighter definition of its core business, with stricter gate keeping, and little attention being devoted to cross-sector collaboration. Hence, the relative isolation of the asylum is replicated in the new psychiatric service system.

The Position of Consumers and Family Carers

Australian mental health policy has emphasised the desirability of participation of consumers and family carers at all levels, from service system design and evaluation to on-the-ground partnership and participation in individual treatment/service plans. For instance the Second National Mental Health Plan introduced, for the first time in a formal sense, the idea that carers as well as consumers had a crucial part to play in the service, rehabilitation and recovery aims of the mental health programmes.

> The range of steps taken to promote consumer and carer participation is one of the hallmarks of the first five years of the National Mental Health Strategy. At the national level, consumers and carers have been included in every planning group established since the Strategy began and considerable funds have been allocated to strengthening their voice in the mental health market place. These initiatives have rippled through to the service delivery field such that these groups now have many more avenues to make their views heard. Arguably, mental health leads the health industry in this area (Commonwealth Department of Health and Aged Care, 2000: 118).

The seminal Deakin workshops (Deakin Human Services Australia, 1999) identified that assessment of the quality of education and training for the National Mental Health Workforce should be based upon two simple but profound guiding principles:

- mental health professionals need to learn about and value the lived experience of consumers and carers
- mental health professionals should recognise and value the healing potential in relationships between consumers and service providers (Deakin Human Services Australia, 1999: 5).

Such principles have had an influence on National Service and Practice Standards in mental health, and there have been other significant changes such as the employment by some services of Consumer and Carer Consultants (employed on a paid basis to represent and advocate for the interests of consumers and carers respectively). Nevertheless, many services remain mysterious and stigmatising, and the potential of consumer and carer participation has yet to be fully realised (Middleton *et al.*, forthcoming). Significantly, attitudes of service providers remain a significant problem, and the view is 'commonly expressed' that 'the mental health workforce itself perpetuates the stigma of mental illness' (Steering Committee for the Evaluation of the Second Mental Health Plan, 1998–2003, 2003: 25; Groom and Hickie, 2003).

A Public Health Approach

The second National Mental Health Plan was the first Australian government mental health document that explicitly built proposals from a base in a public health, population based approach to policy. That is:

> The determinants of physical and mental health status, at the population level, comprise a range of psychosocial and environmental factors including income, employment, poverty, education and access to community resources, as well as demographic factors, most notable gender, age and ethnicity (Commonwealth Department of Health and Aged Care, 2000a).

The third National Mental Health Plan for 2003–2008 continues this emphasis on a whole of community approach (Australian Health Ministers, 2003) and the continuing legitimation of the resultant policy direction of health promotion and prevention. Depression was given some priority as a target disorder in response to the implications of the WHO/World Bank study of the Burden of Disease, which among other things highlighted the rising costs associated with an increasing incidence and prevalence of depression within industrialised countries (Murray and Lopez, 1996; Commonwealth Department of Health and Aged Care and Australian Institute of Health and Welfare, 1999). Solutions canvassed in the promotion and prevention literature include a range of interventions from early case finding, targeted interventions, and community education through to social development. One influential local document, the VicHealth Mental Health Promotion Plan, identifies 'social connectedness', 'freedom from discrimination and violence and economic participation' as the key determinants of mental health and the key organising themes for action (VicHealth, 1999). By contrast mainstream psychiatric views in Australia tend to cite a more limited version of interventions centred around community education as a key measure in reducing the impacts of depression (Jorm, 2000). More particularly *beyondblue: the national depression initiative* has had as its inaugural CEO a Professor of Psychiatry who asserts that:

> Depression prevention is feasible if we focus on providing quality interventions to targeted populations at key moments along the known paths to illness onset or recurrence (Hickie, 2002).

In general the emphasis in practice is upon medical and behavioural change oriented interventions which, while vital to achieving better outcomes for those at risk, are only one part of a more comprehensive social and community building approach to mental health promotion and prevention. The primary mental health teams, which are the public psychiatric service response to prevention, provide support to primary care givers to help them deliver earlier and more effective clinical interventions. In other words the policy implementation leaves little space for community interventions.

Conclusion

The Australian mental health policy processes reflect a complex set of contexts within which the tensions between various ideological and theoretical approaches take on particular meanings and shape service outcomes as they intersect with a range of political and bureaucratic imperatives. As a result the contribution of the psychosocial orientation has had and continues to have a variable impact on how services are constructed and delivered. Nonetheless throughout the system there is evidence of robust debate about and considerable achievements in policy and programme development when factors about whole of life considerations are granted due significance and where the mission of mental health services is understood to be more than merely identifying and treating an illness.

References

Auditor General Victoria (2002), *Mental Health Services for People in Crisis*, Government Printer for the State of Victoria: Melbourne.

Australian Health Ministers (1991), *Mental Health: Statement of Rights and Responsibilities*, Report of the Mental Health Consumer Outcomes Task Force, Australian Government Publishing Service: Canberra.

Australian Health Ministers (1992), *National Mental Health Policy*, Australian Government Publishing Service: Canberra.

Australian Health Ministers (1998), *Second National Mental Health Plan*, Mental Health Branch, Commonwealth Department of Health and Family Services: Canberra.

Australian Health Ministers (2003), *National Mental Health Plan 2003–2008*, Australian Government: Canberra.

Bainbridge, L. (1999), 'Competing paradigms in mental health practice and education', in Pease, B. and Fook, J. (eds), *Transforming Social Work Practice*, Allen and Unwin: Sydney.

Burdekin, B. (2001), *The Age*, Tuesday 31st July.

Carr, V. and Halpin, S. (on behalf of the Low Prevalence Disorders Study Group) (2002), *Stigma and discrimination (Low Prevalence Disorder Component of the National Study of Mental Health and Wellbeing Bulletin No.6*, Commonwealth Department of Health and Ageing: Canberra.

Collison, S. and Copolov, D. (2004), 'Challenges and opportunities for mental health research in Australia', *Journal of Mental Health*, 13, 1, 29-36.

Commonwealth Department of Health and Aged Care and Australian Institute of Health and Welfare (1999), *National Health Priority Areas Report: Mental Health 1998*, Canberra: Australian Institute of Health and Welfare.

Commonwealth Department of Health and Aged Care (2000), *National Mental Health Report 2000: Changes in Australia's Mental Health Services under the First National Mental Health Plan of the National Mental Health Strategy 1993–98*, Australian Government Publishing Services: Canberra.

Commonwealth Department of Health and Aged Care (2000a), *Promotion, Prevention and Early Intervention for Mental Health – A Monograph*, Mental Health and Special Programs Branch, Commonwealth Department of Health and Aged Care: Canberra.

Commonwealth Department of Health and Ageing (2002), *National Mental Health Report 2002: Seventh Report. Changes in Australia's Mental Health under the First Two Years of the Second National Mental Health Plan 1998–2000*, Commonwealth of Australia: Canberra.

Dax, E. (1961), *Asylum to Community*, F.W. Cheshire: Melbourne.

Dax, E. (1992), 'The evolution of community psychiatry', *Australian and New Zealand Journal of Psychiatry*, 26, 295-301.

Deakin Human Services Australia (1999), *Learning Together: Education and Training Partnerships in Mental Health Service Final Report*, National Mental Health Strategy: Canberra.

Dudley, M. (2003), 'Contradictory Australian national policies on self-harm and suicide: The case of asylum seekers in mandatory detention', *Australasian Psychiatry*, 11, Supplement, 102-108.

Groom, G. and Hickie, I. (2003), *Out of Hospital, Out of Mind!: A Review of Mental Health Services in Australia – 2003*, Canberra: Mental Health Council of Australia.

Healy, B. (2002), 'Policy Reform in the Psychiatric Sector: Service Responses after Deinstitutionalisation', in Liamputtong, P and Gardner, H (eds), *Health, Social Policy and Communities*, Oxford University Press: Melbourne.

Healy, B. and Brophy, L. (2002), 'The Law and Psychiatry', in Swain, P. (ed.), *In the Shadow of the Law*, 2nd edn., Federation Press: Melbourne.

Healy, B. and Varney, H. (1995), Mainstreaming and Integrating Psychiatric Services: The Victorian Experience, *Australian Journal of Social Issues*, 130: 2, 179-194.

Hickie, I. (2002), 'Preventing depression: A challenge for the Australian community', *Medical Journal of Australia*, 177, Supplement: 85-86.

Human Rights and Equal Opportunity Commission (1993), *Report of the National Inquiry into the Human Rights of People with Mental Illness*, vols 1 and 2, Australian Government Publishing Service: Canberra.

Hunter, E. and Tsey, K. (2003), 'Setting strategic directions in mental health policy and practice: The challenge of understanding and addressing the social determinants', *Australasian Psychiatry*, 11, Supplement, 1-5.

Hunter, E. and Walter, G. (eds) (2003), Supplement, *Australasian Psychiatry*, 11.

Jablensky, J., McGrath, J., Herrman, H., Castle, D., Gureje, O., Morgan, V. and Korten, A. (1999), *People Living with Psychotic Illness: An Australian Study 1997–98. An Overview*, Mental Health Branch, Commonwealth Department of Health and Aged Care: Canberra.

Jorm, A. (2000), 'Mental health literacy: Public knowledge and beliefs about mental disorders', *British Journal of Psychiatry*, 177, 396-401.

Murray, C.J.L. and Lopez, A.D. (1996), *The Global Burden of Disease*, World Health Organization, Harvard School of Public Health, World Bank: Geneva.

Middleton, P., Stanton, P. and Renouf, N. (2004), 'Consumer Consultants in mental health services: Addressing the challenges', *Journal of Mental Health*, 13, 507-518.

Meadows, G. and Singh, B. (eds) (2001), *Mental Health in Australia: Collaborative Community Practice*, Oxford University Press: Melbourne.

National Mental Health Strategy Evaluation Steering Committee for the Australian Health Ministers Advisory Council (1997), *Evaluation of the National Mental Health Strategy: Final Report*, Canberra: Mental Health Branch, Commonwealth Department of Health and Family Services.

Psychiatric Services Division, Victorian Department of Health and Community Services (1994), *Victoria's Mental Health Service: The Framework for Service Delivery*. Melbourne: Department of Health and Community Services.

Rees, S. (2003), 'Refuge or retrauma? The impact of asylum seeker status on the wellbeing of East Timorese women asylum seekers residing in the Australian community', *Australasian Psychiatry*, 11, Supplement, 96-101.

Steering Committee for the Evaluation of the Second Mental Health Plan 1998–2003 (2003), *Evaluation of the Second National Mental Health Plan*, Canberra: Commonwealth Department of Health and Ageing.

VicHealth (1999), *Mental Health Promotion Plan Foundation Document: 1999–2002*, VicHealth: Melbourne.

Victorian Government Department of Human Services A, Community and Mental Health Division (1998), *Individual Service Planning*, Melbourne: Victorian Government Department of Human Services, Aged, Community and Mental Health Division.

Whiteford, H., Buckingham, B. and Manderscheid, R. (2002), 'Australia's National Mental Health Strategy', *British Journal of Psychiatry*, 180, 210-215.

Zifcak, S. (1996), 'The United Nations principles for the protection of people with mental illness: Applications and limitations', *Psychiatry, Psychology and the Law*, 3, 1-9.

Chapter 4

Contextualised Social Policy: Agenda and Priorities – a UK Perspective

Pauline M. Prior

Introduction

We are at a moment of radical change in mental health law and policy direction throughout Europe, a pattern that is demonstrated clearly in the United Kingdom (UK). Having closed many large psychiatric hospitals, the two-fold task still remains a priority on the health agenda – that of caring for individuals with mental health problems while protecting the public from undue risk. Though the UK consists of three different legal systems – England and Wales, Scotland, Northern Ireland – all legal changes are guided by a single ideology, that of the current government at Westminster. The purpose of this chapter is to focus on the current mental health, policy trends, taking into account the political, legal, professional and social contexts that impinge on them.

Different Agendas

Current UK mental health policies reflect government priorities in relation to public policy on health and on crime, influenced by lobbies from the mental health sector and by other external forces, the most important of which are summarised below.

The Political Agenda

Mental health policy has to be viewed within the context of general social policy as it has emerged under the Labour Government, led by Prime Minister Tony Blair, which replaced the Conservative Government in 1997. Its policies have been characterised by a commitment to the philosophy of the National Health Service (NHS) – the public provision of a health care system, free at the point of delivery and funded from general taxation. Within the framework, Blair promised to modernise mental health services, in terms of both service delivery and legislation. Two policy documents are worth mentioning: 'Modernising Mental Health Services' (DH, 1998), and 'Reforming the Mental Health Act' (DH, 1999).

In 'Modernising Mental Health Services' (DH, 1998), the Government promised:

- To modernise mental health services by providing 'safe, sound and supportive' services.
- To enable 24-hour access to service, ensure public safety and manage risk more effectively.
- To involve patients, service users and carers in their own care and in planning services.
- To integrate mental health services more firmly into primary care services.
- To work in partnership with education, employment and housing.

In 'Reforming the Mental Health Act' (DH, 1999), the Government promised:

- To draw up new legislation that will form part of new arrangements for improving the quality and consistency of health and social services for people who suffer from mental health problems.
- To provide a new structure for the application of compulsory powers of detention for assessment and treatment for the small minority of those who pose a serious threat to the safety of others as a result of their mental disorder.

It is clear from these documents that policy directions in mental health care do not necessarily follow those in physical health care, although this is not always clear to the health professionals working in the mental health care system. In fact, they often reflect policies in relation to crime, based on issues of law and order. The tensions within mental health policy – between the influence of health policy and the influence of law and order policies – are clear in current debates in the UK. While the impetus towards a partnership-model of provision and a community-care model of treatment and care comes directly from the health lobby within government, the impetus towards a risk-avoidance and public-safety strategy comes from the law-and-order lobby. Many mental health professionals and service-users find it difficult to accept the prominent position given to this latter approach in the debate on mental health law and wonder if money will be invested in the services geared towards safety of the public to the detriment of services geared towards care and treatment of service users.

The Human Rights Agenda

Under the European Convention of Human Rights, people with a mental illness, like other citizens, can expect to be protected from arbitrary or unnecessary government interference in their lives. The extra component in relation to this group of people is the fact that national governments are obliged to offer special protection to individuals, who are (for whatever reason) not capable of protecting themselves (see CE, 1999; EC, 1996). Until recently, when the Human Rights Act

1998 came into force, the UK, like many other countries, did not have national legislation, so the only option open to people was to use the *European Court of Human Rights* (ECHR) to challenge their own government either for non-protection or for infringement of rights. In spite of the fact that some of the assumptions, which underpin the perspective on mental illness in the Convention on Human Rights, are outmoded (it was drawn up in 1954) progress has been made on the protection of rights

Some of the rights that have received prominence in cases brought to the ECHR by people with mental illnesses include the right to privacy, the right to a fair hearing within a reasonable time, the right of those detained to medical assessment and review and, finally, the right to family life (for further discussion, see Prior, 2001 and 2003). As an example of the impact of some of these cases on the law and procedures at national level, we look briefly at cases taken by parents with diagnosed mental illnesses who had their children taken into care. On the issue of a right to family life, the ECHR found that though local authorities may have been correct in their decision to take a specific child into care, the process had been such that it had either cut-off or weakened the bond between parents and children in care. Where biological parents cannot offer adequate support to children, statutory authorities may intervene to supply substitute care (see Alston, 1994; Duffy, 1982). This is always a temporary measure in the first instance, as it the duty of welfare authorities to support natural families in fulfilling their parental obligations. This often means facilitating a partner or other adults in the extended family to take on a parenting role, when a parent is not able to cope due to mental health problems. The ECHR has regularly affirmed that the act of taking of a child into public care 'does not necessarily mean that there is no longer any parental right in regard to access' (B. v. the UK, 1987, paragraphs 76-77). When children are temporarily removed from parents who are deemed potentially capable of taking back the care of their children sometime in the future, it is the duty of the authorities to ensure access (which promotes bonding) in order to facilitate a future family life together.

However, in many cases where children remain in care – either with a foster-family or adoptive family – the biological parents feel that they are excluded from any possibility of caring for their children at a future date by the very nature of the arrangements made for access (E.P. v. Italy, 1999; Johansen v. Norway (1), 1996; McMichael v. the UK (1), 1995; Olsson v. Sweden, No. 2, 1992; Olsson v. Sweden, No. 1, 1988; B. v. the UK, 1987; H. v. the UK, 1987). In most of these cases, the authorities were found to be correct in their decision to remove children from parents unable to care for them, but at fault in either banning access (E.P. v. Italy, 1999; Johansen v. Norway (1), 1996) or in making it extremely difficult, for example, through arrangements which placed the children at too great a distance from the parents for frequent visiting to be possible (Olsson v. Sweden, No. 1, 1988).

These cases reflect the fact that a static model of mental health and illness often underpins decisions made by welfare authorities in relation to the care of children. They also show the difficulties involved in ensuring participation by parents with mental health problems in all stages of the decision-making process in relation to the care of their children. This is not always easy, as the disabling effects of a deteriorating state of mental health may prevent a parent from active

tion in the process. The lesson to be learned is that because bureaucratic
cope best with situations that do not change, this adds to the difficulties
experienced by people with mental health problems. All too easily, rights can be
removed for much longer than is necessary, due to a lack of mechanisms for
coping with change or to inertia in organisational structures.

The cases taken to the ECHR show that the human rights of people with
mental illnesses have not been adequately protected by current legislation in most
European countries. The UK is no exception to this, but it is to be hoped that the
human rights agenda is now high on the list of priorities for all of those involved in
reviewing current mental health law in each area of the UK.

Service Users

The overwhelming message from people with mental illnesses is that they find it
extremely difficult to function as full citizens. Rather, they often perceive themselves as
marginalised, stigmatised, and controlled. This situation is compounded by the fact that
there is a higher incidence of diagnosed mental illness among people from
disadvantaged sections of society, leading often to layers of disadvantage (for
discussion, see Middleton and Shaw, 1999; Thornicroft, 1991). Fortunately, there has
been a great expansion in recent years in the number and size of self-help organisations
– groups initiated by existing or former users of psychiatric services, their relatives and
friends. The increase in organisations run by and for service users has been fuelled by a
decrease in mental health services and a loss of faith in the medical model of mental
health care. It has also coincided with a greater awareness of basic human rights and of
citizenship rights by people who had previously taken for granted their exclusion from
many social and economic opportunities (Beresford *et al.*, 1997).

In looking at the range of services provided by user groups, it is clear that
agendas vary. As a general rule, older organisations provide services to support
existing mental health services – day centres, housing projects, leisure projects,
rehabilitation and education. In contrast, newer organisations are much more
influenced by the civil rights movement, and are involved in promoting individual
and group resistance to the status quo. This is carried out largely through advocacy
schemes and lobbying tactics aimed at bringing about changes in policies or
services (for further discussion on specific organisations, see Ramon, 1996). As a
result of the increasing pressures being brought to bear by this expanding user
movement, the rights of individuals who are the recipients of mental health
services, to good quality services and to equality as citizens, are increasingly
debated in policy making circles, as evidenced in their participation in the current
reviews of mental health law taking place throughout the UK.

The Impact of Social Trends

The other major set of influences on current mental health policies in the UK
derive from changes in social structures (including gender relations), demographic
patterns, and in socio-economic trends, some of which are discussed here.

Gender Trends

The experience of mental illness and its treatment are highly gendered (see Hayes and Prior, 2003; Prior, 1999). In the past, women appeared more often than men in psychiatric statistics on morbidity and service use. This was due primarily to the focus in research on depression, anxiety and neurotic disorders, in which women feature more prominently than men. In recent times however, the situation has changed as conditions more often associated with men are included as part of the research design.

In the USA, the large-scale *Epidemiologic Catchment Area* (ECA) study was one of the first to acknowledge substance-dependence and personality disorder as mental conditions in need of professional attention in the same way as depression or anxiety disorders. The ECA found that when these conditions were included in the calculations of psychiatric morbidity, men had a slightly higher overall lifetime prevalence than women for mental disorder (Robins and Regier, 1991: 88, Table 5.3). This was confirmed in another US study – the *National Co-morbidity Study* (NCS), which was specifically aimed at exploring the relationship between substance dependence and recognised mental illnesses. The NCS found men twice as likely as women to have a substance dependence problem – with a lifetime prevalence of almost 36 per cent for men and 18 per cent for women (Kessler *et al.*, 1994: 12). Similar patterns are found in the UK. In the *Psychiatric Morbidity Survey*, men were three times more likely than women to be alcohol dependent and twice as likely to be drug dependent (Jenkins and Meltzer, 1995; Jenkins *et al.*, 1997). In other words, studies of psychiatric morbidity, in which substance abuse and personality disorders are included, show that men are equally if not more vulnerable than women to the experience of a mental health problem.

In relation to the use of mental health services, there is also evidence that there has been a change in gender patterns. While women are higher users of community based mental health services, men seem to be increasingly visible in institution-based care (hospital and residential facility). This seems to be related to the fact that as psychiatric beds decrease and as clinical decisions become increasingly influenced by risk assessments, men are more vulnerable to institutionalisation (Payne, 1996; Prior and Hayes, 2001a, 2001b.). Any mental health service of the future has to take into account the different needs of men and of women in their experience of mental health problems and in their approaches to seeking help. It is clear from recent research that men and women may present differently, but that they are equally in need of mental health services tailored to their needs.

In policy terms, therefore, gender is on the mental health agenda. Not only do we need a system of 'gender proofing' in relation to all mental health policies, but perhaps we need to move towards a more pro-active approach such as that employed in 'gender budgets' in this important area of health policy (for discussion, see the web page of the London Women's Budget Group at www.wbg.org.uk).

Social Exclusion

According to WHO statistics, 1 in 6 people will have some experience of mental ill-health at some time in their lives (see DH, 1998). Whether or not this develops into a serious or a chronic mental illness depends, to a large extent, on the circumstances of the person's life. Evidence shows, for example, that there are much higher levels of diagnosed mental illness among individuals from lower socio-economic groups (Middleton and Shaw, 1999; Thornicroft, 1991). In addition, people from certain ethnic backgrounds seem more vulnerable than others to both the experience of mental illness and to compulsory hospital treatment (Nazroo, 1997; Robins and Regier, 1991; Thornicroft, 1991).

As poverty and social exclusions are unlikely to be eradicated from society, it is clear that people from lower income and socially excluded groups will continue to feature disproportionately in psychiatric statistics. In the UK, these groups will increasingly include people born outside of the UK, due to the fact that migrants (legal and otherwise) form an increasing proportion of the population in poor economic circumstances. Clearly, mental health services in the future need to be culturally appropriate and accessible to people from different ethnic and language groups, a situation which has clear training implications for all mental health professionals (for further discussion on issues of race and inequality in relation to mental health care, see Heller *et al.*, 1996).

An Ageing Population

In common with the rest of the Western industrialised world, the UK has an ageing population. In 1901, about one person in 20 was over the age of 65 and one in 100 was over the age of 75. By 1998 this increased to just over one in six for those over the age of 65 and one in 14 for those over the age of 75. At the same time, the proportion of the population under the age of 16 fell from a third to just over a fifth. Demographic projections suggest that these trends will continue. For example, by 2011, it is predicted that the number of people over the age of 65 will be greater than the number under the age of 16-11.9 million as compared to 11.3 million – and the majority of dependants in the UK will be retired people (ONS, 2000a: 8).

This increase in the older population has been largest among women. Women currently begin to outnumber men from around the age of 50 and by the age of 89 there are about three women to every man in the population. However, the most dramatic gender differences in survival rates have occurred among the 'very old' – people living to the age of 100. In 1911, women centenarians outnumbered men centenarians by about three to one, but by 1996, the rates had increased to eight to one. In other words, for every man who reached the age of 100 in the UK in 1996, there were eight women who had done so. While the number of centenarians is still fairly small – 5,500 in England and Wales in 1996 – the rate of increase since the beginning of the century has been very fast, roughly doubling every decade. Population projections suggest that by 2036, there could be over 40 thousand centenarians alive in England and Wales, the vast majority of whom will be women (ONS, 2000b: 25).

Research has shown that these population changes have had a huge impact on the delivery of health services – including mental health services. Older people are higher users of all types of health services and, in particular, of hospital and residential services. Both men and women feature in these services but, because women live longer, they are beginning to pre-dominate in mental health beds (for discussion see Hayes and Prior, 2003: Chapter 6). Another result has been a review of the law in relation to people in mental health beds (hospitals and residential care facilities). The increasing number of people with dementia or other conditions that affect their capacity to make decisions about their own care, has led to the emergence of a legal instrument to deal with this – the legislation on 'Capacity' or 'Incapacity'. In all three areas of the UK, work is in progress on this. Scotland is in the forefront, with a new law passed in 2000 – *Adults with Incapacity (Scotland) Act*. In England and Wales, the *Mental Incapacity Bill* was published in June 2003 and, in Northern Ireland, a Bill is in preparation.

Throughout the UK, the discussions on proposed changes in mental health law have taken into account the legal discussions on capacity and incapacity. In a word, the hope is that some people who formerly were treated under mental health legislation, even though they did not have a mental illness but lacked capacity, will now be more correctly treated under 'capacity' legislation. This will be less stigmatising and more in keeping with human rights principles. One important spin-off from this might be the introduction of the principle of the right to choose ones representative/next of kin in the event of illness, in the same way as people give 'power of attorney' in the event of loss of capacity.

The Law and Mental Disorder

In the following section, we will focus on the legal changes that have taken place in the past 50 years, moving from the general European scene to the particular situation in the UK.

General Trends

Until the 1960s, most people who were diagnosed as mentally ill and in need of treatment received it in hospital on an involuntary/compulsory basis. Though countries varied in the admission procedures used, most were based on mental health laws initiated in the nineteenth century. These laws had been enacted with a two-fold purpose – firstly, to protect the individual (with a mental illness) from unnecessary or illegal confinement and secondly, to protect society from dangerous people.

Italy was one of the first European countries to publicly declare its abhorrence for a mental health care system that led to segregation and social exclusion. Led by Franco Basaglia, a group of psychiatrists and politicians set up *Psichiatria Democratica* and brought about a radical change in the law. The hope was that large institutions would no longer continue to function, and that compulsory admission to much smaller facilities for treatment would only happen after both a judicial and a medical assessment of the situation (Law 180, enacted in 1978; for discussion see Samele, 1999). Thus, in one swift action, Italy removed the legal basis and the service structure that had deprived so many people of their civil and human rights. All that remained to do was the implementation of the policy.

In countries other than Italy, the process of legal change has been slow. As we begin a new century, the situation is similar in most European countries. The majority of people with diagnosed mental illnesses are treated on a voluntary basis (as with other health services) and most of them live at home or in supported housing projects. Statistics from a study by Reicher-Rossler and Rossler (1993) on involuntary admissions to psychiatric hospitals in Europe, indicated that in 14 countries these admissions formed less than 20 per cent of total admissions. However, there was a wide variation in the statistics, from one per cent in Spain to 50 per cent in Switzerland and Austria and it is clear that the statistics across countries are not entirely comparable due to different criteria being used in gathering the statistics. For example, in some countries, mentally-ill offenders are counted, while in others they are excluded.

However, the statistics do confirm the fact that for a substantial minority of people with mental illness, involuntary treatment in hospital is still a reality – involving the deprivation of liberty and civil rights. For the majority the mental health care system of most countries continues to provide services on a voluntary basis and in the community.

Mental Health Law in the UK

In the UK, current mental health laws date back to the 1980s. In England and Wales, this is the *Mental Health Act 1983*, in Scotland, the *Mental Health (Scotland) Act 1984* and, in Northern Ireland, the *Mental Health (NI) Order 1986*. Since the publication of the White Paper, 'Reforming the Mental Health Act' (DH, 1999), preparation for changes in the law have been underway throughout the UK. As discussed already, there are various interested parties involved in this preparation, all of whom have different priorities and agendas. In each area of the UK, working-parties have been set up by Government to review current laws and to suggest changes. As with capacity/incapacity legislation, Scotland is ahead with new mental health legislation – the *Mental Health (Care and Treatment) Scotland Act 2003*. In England and Wales, a draft *Mental Health Bill*, was published in 2002, while in Northern Ireland, the review of law and services is underway and a Bill in preparation. The *Mental Health Bill* for England and Wales caused serious controversy and, as such, deserves some attention. According to a special report prepared by the Sainsbury Centre for Mental Health, London (SCMH, 2002: 2): 'The Bill is seen by some stakeholders as being too draconian and by others as being impracticable and unworkable'. Though many of the recommended changes are positive, others are not.

Among the positives are the following:

- Expansion of the current advocacy services.
- Enhancement of the Mental Health Review Tribunal system.
- Additional protection for children and for people with organic brain syndrome.
- Increasing emphasis on care plans.

Among the proposals on which there is disagreement (see SCHMH, 2003: 2):

- The introduction of compulsory treatment in the community.
- The introduction of treatment orders that seem to allow transfer of patients from community to prison without independent review.
- The abolition of the current Mental Health Act Commission (its functions to be subsumed into the Health Care Inspectorate).

The most controversial proposal of all has been that relating to compulsory treatment in the community. While many people are not against it in principle, many fear that it should only be introduced if safeguards are in place for the delivery of high quality services to people whose human rights are protected sufficiently. If it leads to further stigmatisation or to a lowering of service take-up, then it would be a retrospective step. The minister responsible for mental health, Ms. Rosie Winterton, has just announced on 8th September 2004 that this measure is to be retained in the legislation (Carvel, 2004).

The other two proposals are also seen as likely to lead to a worsening of services for people with mental health problems rather than to improvements in care.

Concluding Remarks

In this chapter, we have looked at the context of current policy changes in relation to mental health services in the UK. This context includes competing demands from a number of different quarters, demands that have to be integrated into the philosophy underlying any change in the law and direction of services. These demands include international standards of human rights and of transparent justice, national demands for good quality services based on NHS principles, local demand for a safe environment and protection from danger, and individual demands for access to mental health care that will have a positive effect on life.

Scotland has already made the legislative leap by introducing a new mental health law and a new 'incapacity' law. England and Wales, and Northern Ireland are in the process of doing the same. It remains to be seen whether or not the raft of legislative changes leads to more 'care' or more 'control' of people with mental health problems. It also remains to be seen, if mental health services in the future will continue to be dominated by a medical model of care and if this model will be build on a conceptual model of a psychosocial understanding of mental health and illness.

References

Alston, P. (ed.) (1994), *The Best Interest of the Child: Reconciling Culture and Human Rights*, Oxford, Oxford University Press.

Beresford, P., Stalker, K. and Wilson, A. (1997), *Speaking for Ourselves: A Bibliography*, London: Open Services Project, in association with the Social Work Research Centre, University of Stirling.

Carvel, J. (2004), 'Psychiatrists condemn draft mental health bill', *The Guardian*, 9 September, p. 8.

CE (1999), *Recommendation of the Committee of Ministers on Principles Concerning the Legal Protection of Incapable Adults*, Strasbourg: Council of Europe Press (CE 99.5).

DH (1998), *Modernising Mental Health Services*, White Paper. London: Department of Health. Also available at website: www.doh.gov.uk.

DH (1999), *Reforming the Mental Health Act*, White Paper, London: Department of Health. Also available at website: www.doh.gov.uk.

Duffy, P.J. (1982), 'The Protection of Privacy, Family Life and Other Rights under Article 8 of the European Convention on Human Rights', *Year-book of European Law*, 2: 191-238.

EC (1996), 'A new European Disability Strategy' (Draft resolution on equality of opportunity for people with disabilities), Luxembourg: Office for Official Publications of the European Communities. COM (96) 406 final. (Brussels 30.7.1996).

Hayes, B.C. and Prior, P.M. (2003), *Gender and Health Care in the UK: Exploring the Stereotypes*, Basingstoke and New York: Palgrave-Macmillan.

Heller, T., Reynolds, J., Gomm, R., Muston, R. and S. Pattison (1996), *Mental Health Matters*, Basingstoke: Macmillan Press.

Hill, M. (1997), *The Policy Process in the Modern State*, London: Prentice Hall/Harvester Wheatsheaf (3rd edition).

Jenkins, R. and Meltzer, H. (1995), The National Survey of Psychiatric Morbidity in Great Britain, *Social Psychiatry and Psychiatric Epidemiology*, 30: 1-4.

Jenkins, R., Lewis, G., Bebbington, P., Brugha, T,. Farrell, M., Gill, B. and Meltzer, H. (1997), 'The National Psychiatric Morbidity Surveys of Great Britain – Initial Findings from the Household Survey', *Psychological Medicine*, 27: 775-89.

Kessler, R., Mc Gonigle, K., Zhao, S., Nelson, C., Hughes, M., Eshleman, S., Wittchen, H. and Kendler, K. (1994), 'Lifetime and 12 Month Prevalence of DSM-III-R Psychiatric Disorders in the United States. Results from the National Comorbidity Survey', *Archives of General Psychiatry*, 51: 8-19.

Middeton, H. and Shaw, I. (1999), 'Inequalities in Mental Health: Models and Explanations', *Policy and Politics*, 27(1): 43-56.

Nazroo, J. (1997), *Ethnicity and Mental Health*, London: Policy Studies Institute.

ONS (2000a), *Population Trends*, London: The Stationary Office. Spring.

ONS (2000b), *Social Trends*, London: The Stationary Office. Vol. 30.

Payne, S. (1996), 'Masculinity and the Redundant Male: Explaining the Increasing Incarceration of Young Men', *Social and Legal Studies*, 5(2): 159-78.

Prior, P.M. (1999), *Gender and Mental Health*, London: Macmillan.

Prior, P.M. (2001), 'Protective Europe: Does it Exist for People with Mental Illnesses?', *Journal of European Social Policy*, 11(2): 25-38.

Prior, P.M. (2003), 'Removing children from the care of adults with diagnosed mental illnesses – a clash of human rights?', *European Journal of Social Work*, 6(2): 179-190.

Prior, P.M. and Hayes, B.C. (2001a), 'Changing Places: Men Replace Women in Mental Health Beds in Britain', *Social Policy and Administration*, 35(4): 397-410.

Prior, P.M. and Hayes, B.C. (2001b), 'Gender Trends in Occupancy Rates in Mental Health Beds in Northern Ireland', *Social Science and Medicine*, 52: 537-545.

Ramon, S. (1996), *Mental Health in Europe*, London: Macmillan.

Reicher-Rossler, A. and Rossler, W. (1993), 'Compulsory Admission of Psychiatric Patients – An International Comparison (Review Article)', *Acta Psychiatrica Scandinavica*, 87: 231-236.

Robins, L. and Regier, D. (eds) (1991), *Psychiatric Disorders in America*, New York: Free Press.

SCMH (2002), *An Executive Briefing on the Draft Mental Health Bill*, London: Sainsbury Centre for Mental Health.

Thornicroft, G. (1991), 'Social Deprivation and Rates of Treated Mental Disorder', *British Journal of Psychiatry*, 158: 475-84.

Cases Cited – European Court of Human Rights

B. v. the UK. Case No. 5/1986/103/151.Application No. 9840/82. Judgment 25.6.1987

E.P. v. Italy. Application No. 31127/96. Judgment 16.11.1999, (no case number).

H. v. the UK. Case No 3/1986/101/149. Application No. 9580/81. Judgment 26.5.1987.

Johansen v. Norway (1). Case No 24/1995/530/616. Application No. 17383/90. Judgment 27.6.1996.

McMichael v. the UK (1). Case No.51/1993/446/525. Application No.16424/90. Judgment 25.1.1995

Olsson v. Sweden (No.1). Case No. 2/1987/125/176. Application No. 10465/83. Judgment 25.2.1988.

Olsson v. Sweden (No. 2.). Case No 74/1991/326/398. Application No. 13441/87. Judgment 30.10.1992.

For final reports see the web page of the ECHR, http://www.echr.coe.int.

Part Three
Paradigm Shift:
Processes and Outcomes

Chapter 5

Paradigm Shift in Psychiatry

Duncan Double

A recent statement from the American Psychiatric Association (APA, 2003) on the diagnosis and treatment of mental disorders maintained that schizophrenia and other mental disorders are serious neurobiological disorders. This unequivocal stance was made in response to a hunger strike by six survivors of the psychiatric system (Mind Freedom, 2004). The challenge of the hunger strikers was that the APA should provide evidence to show that major mental illnesses are 'proven biological diseases of the brain' and that emotional distress results from 'chemical imbalances' in the brain.

The APA supported its contention of the neurobiological nature of mental illness by claiming that (a) research has shown reproducible abnormalities of brain structure and function (b) evidence for a strong genetic component of mental disorders is compelling, and (c) the mechanisms of action of effective medications have been elucidated. Each of these claims is controversial and the evidence for them can be questioned (Double, 2004).

Why does the position of the APA on mental disorders instigate an extreme reaction such as a hunger strike? This is what I want to look at in this chapter. My thesis is that mainstream psychiatry, represented by the APA, has become contingent on the biomedical model of mental illness. This approach is now so dominant that it seems that any challenge needs to be made by extravagant action.

Although the somatic model of mental illness may have always dominated psychiatric practice, there have been times when psychiatry has been more open to other possibilities. Previously the biological hypothesis would have been recognised as a hypothesis; now it tends to be regarded as fact. Such a consequence may be justified, as in the APA statement, by apparent scientific advances over recent years in the understanding of the neurobiological basis of mental illness. This progress is said to have occurred at the level of neurochemistry by demonstrating the basis of action of psychotropic medications, and at the level of structural and functional abnormalities by the development of brain scanning technology. But is this really the case? Has psychiatry advanced to such a state that the biomedical model is now impregnable?

I don't think so. Instead I want to argue that the controversy is about the most appropriate paradigm for psychiatry. To simplify I want to concentrate on what it might mean to shift from the current, dominant biomedical model to a biopsychological model. Simplification may be necessary when talking about change at the level of paradigm. Inevitably we are trying to distil patterns about the way we view psychiatry. In the real world, people do not always stick very closely to the described model, and there may be variations within one perspective without being totally clear about what constitutes the essence of the approach. Still, I think there is enough agreement about the nature of the biomedical and biopsychological models of mental illness for our discourse to be meaningful. I will use definitions that have clearly stated propositions.

The biopsychological model is not new. For example, it was promoted on the basis of systems theory when such thinking was favoured (Engel, 1977). In many ways, the best representative of the perspective was the Psychobiology of Adolf Meyer (1866–1950) (Winters, 1951/2). Meyer, an immigrant to the United States from Switzerland, had an important role in American psychiatry. He vies to be the foremost American psychiatrist of the first half of the 20th century. Although he lived in the United States for many years, Meyer had a rather convoluted style of communication in English. His ideas never really took hold as a systematic theory of psychiatry (O'Neill, 1980), and maybe for this reason they are now little known.

What I am suggesting is that Meyer's ideas should be better known. Of course, the biopsychological approach has a set of assumptions, concepts, values and practices, as does the biomedical model. I want to look at these assumptions. I also want to look at the natural tendency to favour a biomedical perspective. I want to emphasise that the way we view the reality of mental illness does have ethical consequences.

My discussion will be set in the context of so-called 'anti-psychiatry', a term used for a diverse set of critiques in the 1960s and 70s of the theoretical basis and practice of psychiatry (Tantam, 1991). In particular, I relate a previous shift of paradigm from a biopsychological to a biomedical perspective that occurred about 1970, perhaps particularly in the USA, to the reaction of orthodox psychiatry to the critique of anti-psychiatry. As I said previously, biomedical psychiatry has not always been quite so dominant. There was a retraction of the generally accepted view of psychiatry towards a biomedical bias following the critique of anti-psychiatry. If we can understand what led to this paradigm shift, we may be able to appreciate what needs to happen to reverse it and create a new synthesis.

The neo-Kraepelinian Approach

I want to take what has been called the 'neo-Kraepelinian' approach as the modern expression of the biomedical perspective. Klerman (1977) first enunciated the principles underlying this approach. There are nine propositions, not all entirely discrete from each other. I will briefly look at them each in turn:

(i) *Psychiatry is a branch of medicine*

This is a clear statement about the relationship between psychiatry and the rest of medicine. In many ways, it arises because psychiatry wants to gain the respect of the rest of medicine, rather than be seen as a vague discipline with less authority. It also has implications for non-medical practitioners who are viewed as subsidiary to the appropriate psychiatric professional, i.e. the medical doctor.

(ii) *Psychiatry should use modern scientific methods and base its practice on scientific knowledge*

Science is not defined in this statement. What is implied is natural science, in the sense of causal laws that have been enormously successful in producing technological advances. Placing an emphasis on this objectivity and progress is therefore understandable. Empirical, verifiable, reproducible knowledge is valued for its predictive abilities. The consequence is that 'soft' sciences such as psychoanalysis are viewed as unscientific and unverifiable, although Freud himself regarded psychoanalysis as a deterministic science.

(iii) *Psychiatry treats people who are sick and need treatment for mental illness*

The claim here is that mental illness is like physical illness and people who suffer with mental illness need medical management. The implications for the role of people identified as sick are that they are exempted from responsibility and care needs to be taken of them (Parsons, 1952).

(iv) *A boundary exists between normal and sick people*

An absolute distinction between normality and mental illness is proposed. The implication is that mental illness is foreign to normal experience and therefore attempts to understand its psychogenic origins are discouraged or at least not given priority.

(v) *Mental illness is not a myth; there are many mental illnesses. It is the task of scientific psychiatry to investigate the causes, diagnosis, and treatment of these mental illnesses*

Mental illness is not regarded as a unitary concept in this statement. Discrete mental illnesses are said to be diagnosable with implications for how they are treated. The specific reference to mental illness not being a myth is to counteract the polemic of Thomas Szasz (1972). Szasz regards the concept of mental illness as a category error, because, in his view, the word 'illness' can only be applied to physical disorder and the physical aetiology of so-called 'mental illness' has not been proven. In contrast, neo-Kraepelinianism accepts the somatic hypothesis and advocates more research to elucidate its basis.

(vi) *The focus of psychiatric physicians should be particularly on the biological aspects of mental illness*

We started the chapter with the APA claim that mental illnesses are neurobiological disorders. This claim follows directly from this neo-Kraepelinian proposition. The danger is that focusing too much on the brain as an organ overlooks the experience of the patient as a person.

(vii) *There should be an explicit and intentional concern with diagnosis and classification*

Modern psychiatry concentrates on classification systems such as the International Classification of Disease now in its 10th edition (ICD-10) (World Health Organisation, 1992) and the Diagnostic and Statistical Manual of the American Psychiatric Association (1994), now in its fourth edition (DSM-IV). From this perspective, the aim of clinical assessment is to identify 'the' diagnosis. The problem is that a false impression of knowledge may be created by a single word diagnosis that reifies the complexity of people's problems.

(viii) *Diagnostic criteria should be codified, and a legitimate and valued area of research should be to validate such criteria by various techniques. Psychiatry departments in medical schools should teach these criteria and not belittle them, as has been the case for many years*

Operational criteria of psychiatric disorders were introduced following the original paper by Feighner *et al.* (1972). Symptom checklists and formal decision-making rules for diagnoses were produced. This trend was followed with the introduction of DSM-III. The aim was to improve the reliability of psychiatric criteria, so that they could be applied more consistently (Spitzer and Fleiss, 1974). The reference to belittling of criteria refers to the Meyerian approach to diagnosis, which saw the understanding of the person as more important than the convenience of a nomenclature.

(ix) *Statistical techniques should be used in research efforts directed at improving the reliability and validity of diagnosis and classification*

Inter-rater reliability can be measured and empirical support for proposed criteria can be obtained in field trials. The concordance of different diagnostic criteria and their coverage can be calculated (Blashfield, 1994). Careful analysis of the evidence presented in reliability studies may not be as much in favour of operational criteria as is commonly assumed (Kutchins and Kirk, 1997). Moreover, low reliability does not necessarily imply poor validity in all contexts, as over precise definitions can be less valid (Carey and Gottesman, 1978).

These nine propositions clearly define the neo-Kraepelinian position. It can be seen as the modern representative of biomedical psychiatry, set in the context of the development of DSM-III and IV. By way of contrast, I want to move on to define the biopsychological perspective.

Biopsychological Approach

As previously mentioned, Adolf Meyer could be seen as the best representative of the biopsychological approach. The essence of his approach was his emphasis on the assessment of the person. Although the mind is contingent on the brain, the central therapeutic concern should be the life story of the individual patient interacting with others in the context of society and culture. Although Meyer introduced Americans to Kraepelin's classificatory system of specific disease entities, he later developed a unitary nosology in which he considered the various classical syndromes to be reaction types (the 'ergasias', from the Greek *ergon*, meaning energy). He stressed the dynamic nature of psychiatric illness, and was opposed to the idea that a hypothetical underlying lesion should be postulated just because mental disorders may seem unintelligible. The assumptions of the biopsychological model are listed by Wilson (1993). Again, I want to look briefly in turn at each of these propositions:

(i) *The boundary between mentally well and mentally ill people is fluid because normal people can become ill if exposed to sufficiently severe trauma*

This proposition is in contrast to the neo-Kraepelinian position that there is an absolute differentiation between normality and mental illness. Instead the relative nature of the continuum between mental illness and normality is emphasised.

(ii) *Mental illness is conceived along a continuum of severity from neurosis through borderline conditions to psychosis*

Again, rather than viewing mental illnesses as discrete entities, as in the neo-Kraepelinian perspective, the emphasis is on the overlap between the various presentations of mental disorder.

(iii) *An untoward mixture of noxious environment and psychic conflict causes mental illness*

Psychosocial factors predominate in the understanding of the aetiology of functional mental illness. For example, Meyer (1906) explained schizophrenia (dementia praecox) as a maladaptation that could be understood in terms of the patient's life experiences. Although psychotic phenomena may seem 'un-understandable' (Jaspers, 1963), efforts need to be made to make sense of such experiences. It is not necessary to postulate a brain abnormality merely because of the difficulty in elucidating the psychosocial context of mental illness.

(iv) *The mechanisms by which mental illness emerges in an individual are psychologically mediated*

The emphasis is on the understanding of human action rather than a reductive analysis of physical causes. A single-word diagnosis may not help much to explain the mechanism of mental illness.

Again, these propositions provide a clear definition of the biopsychological perspective. Having stated our definitions, I want to move on to a comparison of the foundations of the two approaches. I want to analyse why there tends to be a bias in favour of the biomedical rather than biopsychological model.

Comparison of the Idea of Mental Illness from Biopsychological and Biomedical Perspectives

The conceptual foundations of Meyer's Psychobiology are different from those of neo-Kraepelinianism. Essentially, the differences could be said to relate to how the two approaches attempt to answer two main philosophical issues (a) the mind-body problem and (b) the application of scientific method to the study of human nature. In looking at these two problems, which are not totally unrelated, I also want to look at some reasons why biomedical solutions may be favoured over the biopsychological.

(a) *The Mind-body Problem*

The paradox of the mind-body split is exposed in the dichotomy between the subjectivity of mind and the causal laws of matter and motion. By contrast, Meyer argued for mind-brain integration, bringing the mind and body together in his concept of Psychobiology. He wanted to avoid a dualistic solution, such as Cartesianism. In particular he wanted to move on from the 'doctrine of psychophysical parallelism', which views mental and physical events as occurring in parallel.

The biomedical model comes to a different solution and instead focuses on the brain as the cause of mental illness. Mind then tends to be seen as secondary or an epiphenomenon of physiological and other physical processes. The speculation is that abnormalities at a biological level will be demonstrated to explain mental illness. Although the hypothetical nature of the disease basis of mental illness may be acknowledged, there are clearly strong factors encouraging the step of faith in the hypothesis. The physical world is seen as objective and more substantial compared to the subjectivity and insubstantiality of mind. The factors favouring objectivity must be powerful as it could be said to leave us without knowledge of what really matters, which is meaningful existence in the world.

How does avoiding the personal dimension then help? Let us look at an example of the potential advantage. This element is related to the notion of responsibility and blame for mental disorder. A biomedical perspective, because it looks for the explanation in the brain, could be seen as avoiding such niceties. For instance, Anthony Clare (1997) has condemned the cultural critique of psychiatry by R.D. Laing. In Clare's words:

> Many parents of sufferers from schizophrenia cannot forgive [Laing] … for adding the guilt of having 'caused' the illness in the first place to their strains and stresses of having to be the main providers of support.

This seems to be an overarching reason why Laing should be dismissed. It is actually a misunderstanding of his views. One only has to read *The Politics of Experience*, commonly regarded as the most 'radical' of Laing's books to find a clear quote that counters this perception:

> [It is not] a matter of laying blame at anyone's door. The untenable position, the 'can't win' double-bind, the situation of checkmate, is by definition *not obvious* to the protagonists (Laing, 1967: 95).

Laing is not talking about conscious motivation to cause harm. He took an interest in Sartre's concept of dialectical rationality and translated Sartre's work with David Cooper in the book *Reason and Violence* (Laing and Cooper, 1964). He would not have been so naive as to suggest that what he was proposing was a causal one-to-one connection between schizophrenia and the family. This misinterpretation of Laing has discouraged further study of the family context of mental illness. Instead, the myth is perpetuated that a biopsychological critique, such as Laing's, leads to unnecessary and unfair criticism of the influence of the family in the causation of schizophrenia. Focusing on the brain rather than family context seems to avoid this dilemma.

A more recent example of the same phenomenon, demonstrating the motivating factor of avoiding blame can be seen in the debate about the validity of attention-deficit/hyperactivity disorder (ADHD) in children. An international consensus statement (Barkley, 2002), essentially arguing that ADHD is not primarily the result of environmental factors, ends with the following sentence:

> ADHD should be depicted ... as a valid disorder having varied and substantial adverse impact on those who may suffer from it through no fault of their own or their parents and teachers.

In other words, the advantage of a neurobiological hypothesis of ADHD is that it creates a neutral physical disorder, taking us out of the realm of personal and social fault and blame for the disorder. I can understand why people may want to avoid these difficult issues. Parents may do dreadful things to their children, not always consciously. Developmental factors are crucial in the behaviour of children. But can we really avoid looking at these reasons for human action?

As in the case of Laing, it is a mistake to suggest that cultural critics of the biomedical model of ADHD are primarily motivated by the wish to attribute blame. The biopsychological perspective is merely suggesting that consideration of personal, family and social factors is important. This analysis needs to be undertaken before moving on to think about blame and responsibility.

(b) *The Importance of the Scientific Method*

The other aspect of the conceptual foundations of understanding mental illness that I want to consider is concerned with the role of science. Scientific abstractions about physical processes have been enormously successful. How mind becomes an object for scientific study is more open for debate. Biopsychological and biomedical perspectives take different views on this issue.

Meyer, as the representative of the biopsychological model, had a broad notion of science that included the study of the person. He took over the Huxleyan notion of science as being 'organised commonsense'. As far as he was concerned, science not only has a physical basis but also can be applied to mental life.

By contrast, biomedical psychiatry is positivist in the sense that the purpose of science is regarded as objective observation. Empirical sciences are the only source of true knowledge. Since the origins of modern psychiatric practice, the contention has been that all that is needed is more research to uncover the physical basis of mental illness.

What is it about the biomedical approach that gives it an advantage in this debate? After all, it is not clear how to decide *a priori* between the legitimacy of the biomedical and biopsychological models of mental illness. To obtain an answer to this question, we can look at criticisms of Meyer by biomedical psychiatrists. For example, Slater and Roth (1969) regarded the Meyerian approach as 'almost entirely sterile'. What they meant by this was that Meyer seemed to foreclose discussion at too vague a level. Meyer realised that attempting to understand mental disorder at the personal level did not necessarily provide dependable and effective data and that it could be 'scoffed at' for this reason. Biomedical science seems to hold out the possibility of certainty and this factor does sway heavily in the debate.

For example, we can look at the views of John Haslam (1764–1844), apothecary at Bedlam during 1792–1815 (Scull *et al.*, 1996). Using him as our example shows that the psychological pressures to believe in the biological hypothesis of mental illness are not new. For example, in his book *Considerations on the moral management of insane persons* (1817) he concluded that insanity is 'a corporeal disease'. The professional implications for him were clear, because it then made mental illness 'the peculiar and exclusive province of the *medical* practitioner' (his emphasis). His motivation to reach this conclusion is disclosed another book *Observations on insanity* (1798):

> [T]he various and discordant opinions, which have prevailed in this department of knowledge, have led me to disentangle myself as quickly as possible from the perplexity of metaphysical mazes.

In other words, he was taking a positivist perspective of mental illness, in which metaphysical aspects of mind related to meaning are just too complex for him to be concerned with. Notwithstanding intuitive understanding of mental illness as a disorder of the mind, it is simpler to concentrate on its bodily substrate. Ironically, as he himself said, '[F]rom the limited nature of my powers, I have never been able to conceive ... *a disease of the mind*' (again his emphasis). A disease of the brain provides a firmer foundation than the woolly notion of psychological abnormality.

I can understand the craving for logical unity and simplicity. However, the reality is that human action is complex and ultimately unpredictable for individuals. Application of the scientific method to human behaviour may hold out the possibility of absolute conditions, but we may nonetheless continue to have to struggle with the relative nature and ethical dimension of our practice in psychiatry.

The Social Dimension of Mental Illness

The advantage of the biopsychological model is that it encourages an emphasis on context and therefore brings a social dimension to the understanding of mental illness. Before moving on to discuss the nature of the paradigm shift between biomedical and biopsychological perspectives, I want to make some comments about this social dimension.

Laing's views about the family, which we have already mentioned, clearly provide this perspective. *The politics of the family* (Laing, 1971) reinforced the importance of understanding people in social situations. Laing saw himself as a psychiatrist commonly being called into a social crisis defined as a medical emergency.

Laing gives examples of how situations need to be uncovered. Rather than constructing situations in terms of psychiatric 'myths', an effort needs to be made to make sense of people's stories. For Laing, few psychiatrists are experts in sorting out these stories.

The implication for service users and their families is that the biopsychological approach avoids making too much of a single word biomedical diagnosis (Double, 2002). Their complex problems are not reified into an hypothesised biological abnormality. If no physical lesion is postulated, there is less emphasis on physical treatments, such as medication.

The social dimension is crucial, but it is important not to seek a total explanation in social terms for mental illness, which is essentially psychological rather than social dysfunction. As an example, I want to consider the notion of mental illness as social deviance. This is just one of a number of aspects of the social dimension of mental health and illness. Others include social structural issues, such as social class, poverty, oppression, social exclusion and injustice, which may be implicated in the sequences of events leading to mental health problems. Other research looks for explanatory associations with various psychosocial dimensions and life events. For example, the study by Brown and Harris (1978) into depression in women implicated vulnerability factors such having three children under the age of 14 years, not working outside the home, having no one to confide in and loss of one's mother by death or separation before the age of 11 years.

Labelling theory is a particularly influential social theory of mental illness. This theory is perhaps most closely associated with the name of Thomas Scheff. His classic 1966 textbook has been reissued and there have been significant mollifying differences in the argument from the first edition (Scheff, 1999).

The mentally ill person does not fit into society and can therefore be seen as deviant. The essential point of Scheff's theory is that the person perceived as mentally ill is the deviant for which society does *not* provide an explicit label. Of all the categories of norm violations, such as crime, perversion, drunkenness and bad manners, labelling someone as mentally ill is identified as *residual* rule-breaking.

Scheff's theory proposes that stereotyped imagery of mental disorder is learnt in early childhood and is continually reaffirmed, inadvertently, in ordinary social interaction and in the mass media. Labelled deviants may be rewarded by doctors and others for conforming to the idea of how a patient ought to behave when ill. They may be systematically blocked from returning to the non-deviant role once the label has been applied. Labelling is seen as an important cause of ongoing residual deviance. Labelling theory describes the process of social control – it does not imply intentionality.

Scheff's theory is compatible with wider aspects of 'anti-psychiatry', such as the study of families of schizophrenics by Laing and Esterson (1964). This research describes the disturbed and disturbing patterns of communication that lead to the labelled family member being elected to the role of 'schizophrenic'. For Laing as much as Scheff, the label is a social event and the social event a political act.

Anti-psychiatry, therefore, came to regard psychiatric practice as repressive in that it was seen as identifying and suppressing social dissent. For example, Laing (1967) was explicit that civilisation represses transcendence and so-called 'normality' is too often an abdication of our true potentialities.

Despite the implications of anti-psychiatry, social deviance cannot be the total definition of mental illness (Lewis, 1955). Other forms of deviance, such as criminality, exist in society. It is not always sufficiently appreciated that Scheff's theory could be seen as accommodating this point by proposing that mental illness is residual deviance i.e. his theory acknowledges other forms of deviance.

The problem with labelling theory is that it could be seen as ignoring the individual dimension and, in this sense, overstating the social basis of the theory. Thomas Scheff came to realise that the approach of his original edition was too one dimensional, and did not sufficiently acknowledge the integration of individual and social factors. The theory also tends to avoid social structural issues, such as social class.

Mental illness is primarily a psychological concept, in that it points to abnormalities in psychological functioning (Farrell, 1979). Social deviance itself cannot be used as evidence, let alone sufficient evidence for diagnosing mental illness.

Even if a thoroughgoing sociological explanation of mental illness, in a Durkheimian sense, is unsuccessful, the social nature of psychiatric practice cannot be denied. Labelling theory does need to be taken seriously, as mental health practice is inevitably a form of social control. To be identified as mentally ill implies social maladjustment. Biological psychiatrists may play down any close tie between mental illness and social deviance because they wish to emphasise individual somatic abnormality. However, psychiatric intervention occurs in social context. The environment and milieu cannot be disregarded.

Psychiatry does have a cultural role and is directly related to social control through the Mental Health Act. Historically the practice of psychiatry arose in the asylum. Mental health practice needs to accept this social perspective and, therefore, explicitly place itself in its ethical context. It needs to define its role and responsibilities in relation to human rights, freedom and coercion. How we understand mental illness does make a difference.

Paradigm Shift Between Biomedical and Biopsychological Perspectives

Let us summarise where we have got to in our account of paradigmatic understanding of mental illness. To simplify, we have concentrated on biomedical and biopsychological perspectives. We have looked at definitions of these two positions and the various propositions underlying them. We then discussed the conceptual foundations of the two approaches, not in an exhaustive way, but so that we can appreciate illustrations of how and why the biomedical perspective becomes favoured. We acknowledged that the social dimension cannot, and should not, be ignored.

I now want to move on to look at the paradigmatic shift that occurred in mainstream psychiatry following the critique of anti-psychiatry. Finally, I want to put this change into the current context of psychiatric practice. We need to understand the barriers to any shift back to a biopsychological paradigm. Any hope of a shift in this direction may be unrealistic.

(a) *From Biopsychological to Biomedical*

In retrospect, the view that mental illnesses have primarily psychological causes could be regarded as a brief interlude in the history of psychiatry, covering no more than the period 1900–1970 (Roth and Kroll, 1986). Psychoanalysis was influential, as well as Meyerian psychobiology, particularly in the USA during this period. These forces became less prevalent as the biological model of mental illness reasserted its dominance following the development of modern psychopharmacology with the introduction of chlorpromazine, the first neuroleptic medication for schizophrenia. In the early years of psychopharmacology, much less than in current practice, there was controversy about whether psychoactive drugs were an advance in treatment.

Under Meyer's influence, American psychiatry came to have a distinctively pragmatic, instrumental and pluralistic approach. In the immediate post-war years,

Karl Menninger's (1963) *The Vital Balance* represented a broadly conceived psychosocial theory of psychopathology. Menninger regarded Meyer's efforts, together with those of William Alanson White, as influential forces in producing a unitary concept of mental illness.

This apparent unanimity was broken by the late 1960s. Psychiatry came under intense attack on a number of different fronts. The anti-psychiatry movement, made up of an ideologically and politically diverse group of critics, ranging from the radical libertarian views of Thomas Szasz to the revolutionary critique of self and society by David Cooper, viewed psychiatry as an agent of social control. What these critiques have in common is the sense that psychiatry itself is part of the problem by its objectification of those diagnosed as mentally ill (Jones, 1998). Many became sceptical that psychiatry could diagnose and treat patients. The anti-authoritarian, popular, even romantic, appeal of anti-psychiatry produced an array of criticism of the use of psychiatric diagnosis, psychotropic medication, ECT treatment and involuntary hospitalisation.

The response from mainstream psychiatry was to attempt to make psychiatric diagnoses more reliable. From the 1950s there was increasing concern about the reliability of psychiatric diagnoses. Empirical studies of inter-clinician agreement reached disquieting conclusions about the consistency of psychiatric diagnosis. The inherent vagueness in category definitions due to the Meyerian approach was blamed. Although careful analysis of the evidence presented in these reliability studies may not be as negative as this conclusion may suggest, the commitment to increase diagnostic reliability became a goal in itself

This explicit and intentional concern with psychiatric diagnosis was developed following the original paper by Feighner *et al.* (1972). Diagnostic criteria were operationalised by constructing symptom checklists and formal decision-making rules. This trend was followed in the evolution of the Research Diagnostic Criteria (Spitzer *et al.*, 1975) and in work which started in 1974 on the revision of DSM-II, through editions of DSM-III, DSM-IIIR and DSM-IV (American Psychiatric Association, 1994).

Although DSM-III itself may not have been covertly committed to a biological perspective, the increasing evidence base for pharmacological treatment, as well as developments in genetics and brain scanning, led to the biomedical model being regarded as the only valid method of psychiatry (Guze, 1989). There had been a shift from a biopsychological to a biomedical perspective. This emphasis remains today, and can be seen, for example, in the statement from the American Psychiatric Association (2003) with which we started the chapter.

(b) *From Biomedical to Biopsychological?*

Is it possible to shift back from the hegemony of the biomedical model? A problem is that criticism of the biomedical model tends to be viewed as denial of the reality of mental illness. This may be a way of marginalising the impact of the criticism. Debate tends to become polarised. If there is to be a paradigmatic shift back to a biopsychological model, somehow the message must be promulgated that questioning the biological basis of mental disorder does not necessarily amount to denial of the reality of mental illness or invalidation of the practice of psychiatry. We also need to move on from dismissing all criticism of the biomedical model as 'anti-psychiatry'.

In summary, the problem with the claim that mental disorders are biological diseases is that it creates the reductionist tendency to treat people as brains that need their lesions cured. Psychosocial factors in aetiology tend to be avoided. If biological and genetic factors determine psychopathology, the implication may be that personal and social efforts to improve one's state of mind may be pointless. Treating the biological abnormality and not the person, therefore, has ethical implications. To repeat, this critique is not meant to imply that bodily factors can or should be ignored.

Too much is invested in the biomedical model to expect this argument to produce much change. As we have discussed, the biomedical model tends to avoid the personal dimension. An advantage of this strategy is that it protects those trying to provide care from the pain experienced by those needing support. The temptation to retreat into objectification of those identified as mentally ill may be overwhelming.

Furthermore, the biomedical model tends to avoid the uncertainty of human action. Clear prescriptions for treatment may appear to simplify the response to mental suffering. Complexity and uncertainty may make mental health practice too difficult.

I have tended to concentrate on the psychological barriers to acceptance of the biopsychological paradigm. I don't really see these being overcome very easily. However, I would like to see more acceptance of a pluralistic approach to psychiatry. Biomedicine is not the only paradigm. An interpretative, biopsychological approach has as much consensus as the dominant biomedical model. This argument is conceptual. My main aim in this chapter has been to stimulate a professional debate about the ideological basis of psychiatry.

The point of the chapter has been to highlight biomedical bias in psychiatry, rather than provide a full critique. A more systematic analysis would have to cover more areas. For example, materialistic factors maintaining the biomedical perspective, such as the need to support academic research and defend pharmaceutical company profits, would require more space than this chapter allows me.

Nonetheless, however broad brush my argument may have been, I hope I have highlighted the value and strength of a biopsychological perspective in psychiatry. Shift in the currently dominant, biomedical paradigm is necessary, however strong the barriers to change may be.

References

American Psychiatric Association (1994), *Diagnostic and Statistical Manual of Mental Disorders* (4th edition), Washington: American Psychiatric Association.

American Psychiatric Association (2003), *Statement on Diagnosis and Treatment of Mental Disorders*, Release no 03-39, 25 September 2003 (www.psych.org/news_room/press_releases/mentaldisorders0339.pdf).

Barkley, R.A. (2002), 'International consensus statement on ADHD', January 2002, *Clinical Child and Family Psychology Review*, **5**, 89-111.

Blashfield, R.K. (1984), *The Classification of Psychopathology: Neo-Kraepelinian and Quantitative Approaches*, New York: Plenum.

Brown, G.W. and Harris, T. (1978), *Social Origins of Depression*, London: Tavistock.

Carey, G. and Gottesman, I.I. (1978), 'Reliability and validity in binary ratings: Areas of common misunderstanding in diagnosis and symptom ratings', *Archives of General Psychiatry*, 35, 1454-1459.

Clare, A. (1997), in Mullan, B. (ed.) *R.D. Laing: Creative Destroyer*, London: Cassell.

78 *Mental Health at the Crossroads*

Double, D.B. (2002), 'The overemphasis on biomedical diagnosis in psychiatry', *Journal of Critical Psychology, Counselling and Psychotherapy*, 2, 40-47.

Double, D.B. (2004), 'Biomedical bias of the American Psychiatric Association', *Ethical Human Psychology and Psychiatry* [in press] (available at www.criticalpsychiatry.co.uk/biomedicalbias.htm).

Engel, G.L. (1977), 'The need for a new medical model: A challenge for biomedicine', *Science*, 196, 129-136.

Farrell, B.A (1979), 'Mental illness: A conceptual analysis', *Psychological Medicine*, 9, 21-35.

Feighner, J.P., Robins, E., Guze, S.B., Woodruff, R.A., Winokur, G. and Munoz, R. (1972), 'Diagnostic criteria for use in psychiatric research', *Archives of General Psychiatry*, 26, 57-63.

Guze, S. (1989), 'Biological psychiatry: Is there any other kind?', *Psychological Medicine*, 19, 315-323.

Jaspers, K. (1963), *General Psychopathology*, 7th edition. (transl. Hoening, J. and Hamilton, M.W.) Manchester: University Press.

Jones, C. (1998), 'Raising the anti: Jan Foudraine, Ronald Laing and anti-psychiatry', in Gijswijt-Hofstra, M. and Porter, R. (eds), *Cultures of Psychiatry*, Amsterdam: Editions Rodopi, pp. 283-294.

Klerman, G.L. (1978), 'The evolution of a scientific nosology', in Shershow, J.C. (ed.) *Schizophrenia: Science and Practice*, Cambridge, Mass: Harvard University Press.

Kutchins, H. and Kirk, S.A. (1997), *Making us Crazy: DSM: The Psychiatric Bible and the Creation of Mental Disorders*, New York: Free Press.

Laing, R.D. (1967), *The Politics of Experience and The bird of Paradise*, London: Penguin.

Laing, R.D. (1971), *The Politics of the Family and Other Essays*. London: Tavistock.

Laing, R.D. and Cooper, D.G. (1964), *Reason and Violence*, London: Tavistock Publications.

Laing, R.D. and Esterson, A. (1964), *Sanity, Madness and the Family*, London: Tavistock.

Lewis, A. (1955), 'Health as a social concept', *British Journal of Sociology* 4: 109-124.

Menninger, K. (with Mayman, M. and Pruyser, P.) (1963), *The Vital Balance*, New York: The Viking Press.

Meyer, A. (1906), 'Fundamental concepts of dementia praecox', *British Medical Journal*, 2, 757-759.

Mind Freedom (2004), *Fast for freedom in mental health*, www.mindfreedom.org/mindfreedom/hungerstrike.shtml (Accessed 1 March 2004).

O'Neill, J.R. (1980), 'Adolf Meyer and American psychiatry today', *American Journal of Psychiatry*, 137, 460-464.

Parsons, T. (1952), *The Social System*, London: Tavistock.

Roth, M. and Kroll, J. (1986), *The Reality of Mental Illness*, Cambridge: Cambridge University Press.

Scheff, T.J. (1999), *Being Mentally Ill: A Sociological Theory* (Third edition). New York: Aldine de Gruyter.

Scull, A., MacKenzie, C. and Hervey, N. (1996), *Masters of Bedlam: The Transformation of the Mad-Doctoring Trade*, Chichester: Princeton University Press.

Slater, E. and Roth, M. (1969), *Clinical Psychiatry* (Third edition), London: Bailliere, Tindall and Cassell.

Spitzer, R.L. and Fleiss, J.L. (1974), 'A reanalysis of the reliability of psychiatric diagnosis', *British Journal of Psychiatry*, 125, 341-347.

Spizer, R.L., Endicott, J. and Robins, E. (1975), *Research Diagnostic Criteria (RDC) for a Selected Group of Functional Disorders*, New York: New York State Psychiatric Institute.

Szasz, T.S. (1972), *The Myth of Mental Illness*, London: Paladin.

Tantam, D. (1991), 'The anti-psychiatry movement', in Berrios, G.E. and Freeman, H. (eds), *150 Years of British Psychiatry, 1841–1991*, London: Gaskell, pp. 333-347.

Wilson, M. (1993), 'DSM-III and the transformation of American psychiatry: A history', *American Journal of Psychiatry*, 150, 399-410.

Winters, E. (ed.) (1951/2), *The Collected Papers of Adolf Meyer*, Vols 1-4, Baltimore: Johns Hopkins Press.

World Health Organisation (1992), *The ICD-10 Classification of Mental and Behavioural Disorders*, Geneva: WHO.

Chapter 6

Paradigm Shift in Psychiatry: Processes and Outcomes

Roberto Mezzina

The Shift in Mental Health Paradigms: Introduction

It is extremely difficult to define the current framework for psychiatry and mental health. None of the promises of the so-called 'decade of the brain' in the USA, and therefore in the Western world in general, seem to have come about. There have been no decisive discoveries regarding the functioning of the normal brain, let alone the 'pathological' one. There has been no progress beyond the generic recycling of multi-factor models for mental illness, first formulated over 30 years ago (Strauss and Carpenter, 1981; Zubin and Spring, 1977), but without any conjectures on the weight and role of the individual factors (Ciompi, 1983). The mapping of the human genome has yet to produce applications in psychiatry and the various genetic hypotheses, even those which are not absolutely unscientific and concocted ad hoc, such as the investigation into the reproduction of stigmata of vulnerability at the level of communication and language rather than the illness in itself (Crow and Deakin, 1987) have yet to be confirmed.

The neo-positivist illusion, in the form of the medical and especially the biological models, which sought to govern illness by acting upon the symptoms and/or otherwise confining the ill person in extremely restricted spatial-temporal limits, now appears superseded and anachronistic. The apparently simple and economical possibility that human life, from India to Australia, could be modified in a decisive manner by the mere manipulation of a series of neurotransmitters without having to act upon the specific conditions of unhappiness deriving from an individual's personal and social experience, seems to have been largely abandoned, if not discarded entirely.

As Robert Castel (1982) foresaw, this 'new age' in psychiatry involves a downsizing and, at times, a partial superseding of psychiatric hospitals, at least in advanced countries, but not the prohibition of forms of coercion and exclusion, in a difficult balance between the ethical duty to 'cure' patients who are 'unaware' of their condition, and the control of deviancy which society has always demanded of psychiatry. The forms and places for treatment seem to be spread increasingly over a range that extends from the hardcore to the 'soft', with limited discretion other than that imposed by the social status of the patient which spares some the more traumatic experiences and gives some access to more acceptable forms of treatment. At the same time we are witnessing a major pathologisation and medicalisation of normality which spreads to the definitions of the various therapies applied in its name.

However, if considered in its most radical aspects, there can be no doubt that we are witnessing a period marked, to use Thomas Kuhn's phrase, by a 'paradigm shift' in this area (Kuhn, 1962). A paradigm (a set of theoretical assumptions, practices and knowledge transfers) is being challenged not only by the increase in the number of empirical and conceptual anomalies but also by actual practices.

The paradigm shift that is taking place, even if in a confused fashion, is the passage from the biological-medical model for treating illness to a model of responses to a suffering person's real and tangible needs including those which are psychological and highly subjective, or as the sociologists say, post-materialist needs in order to help them in their often long and difficult journey of recovery and, if need be, of emancipation.

A more indirect strategy thus imposes itself, founded on the simple but radical observation that by now the greater part of the life-cycle of a person who suffers from a severe mental disorder takes place outside the institutions. These latter once defined the limits in an inflexible and often permanent manner, sanctioning an exclusion in terms which were truly absolute. Once community is accepted as the new scenario, the challenge will be to demonstrate the ability to adopt practices that are alternatives to total institutions, and which are also functional (Polak and Kirby, 1976; Mosher and Menn, 1977, 1989; Fenton *et al.*, 1998; Ciompi *et al.*, 1992; Moltzen *et al.*, 1986; Dell'Acqua and Cogliati Dezza, 1985; De Leonardis *et al.*, 1986). This means creating *new models of care* which are, if not more effective, then socially and individually more acceptable (Hoult and Reynolds; Hoult *et al.*, 1984; Hoult, 1986; Stein and Test, 1978, 1985; Andrews *et al.*, 1990; Marks *et al.*, 1994; Dean *et al.*, 1993; Mezzina and Vidoni, 1995), and which guarantee a true 'social reproduction' of the individual, even though (or even if) that person is ill.

In a way which unconsciously reproduces the individualistic fragmentation and solitude of the globalised individual (Baumann, 2000), the new innovative experiences are paying the price of naively presenting models in terms of an absolute efficacy which is uprooted from the historical and local conditions which produced them.

But can we speak of a new, world-wide model which is emerging from this crisis? What elements do the various experiences for change have in common, beyond their unique characteristics, which are contingent upon specific historical and geographical conditions and circumstances (Rosen *et al.*, 1997)? Are the new alternative community-based practices about to arrive at a critical mass, resulting in something which can be considered a trend (IMHCN, 2001)?

The existence of a scientific status for psychiatry has been challenged by a whole stream of Western thought which is critical of objective sciences applied to human beings and by an historical analysis of the roots of psychiatry itself (Sartre, 1960; Goffmann, 1961; Husserl, 1970; Deleuze and Guattari, 1972; Foucault, 1972; Castel, 1976; Porter, 1987). It partially influenced the critical movement toward psychiatric institutions which resulted in de-institutionalisation (Laing, 1968; Jones, 1974; Basaglia, 1987; Tosquelles, 1992).

Psychiatric knowledge has always been produced and modified through a dialectic process with the existing institutions (Basaglia, 1987c). This process confirms, legitimises and supersedes them but also conceals the form of that knowledge. Therapeutic practices have been crystallised into forms which, at any given moment, become fixed and reified, susceptible only to partial change because they are implemented into the unchanging setting (and culture) that emerged basically from the asylum (Basaglia, 1987b). In other words, the asylum provided the ultimate rationale, cultural background and thus the meaning for those practices (De Leonardis *et al.*, 1986; Rotelli, 1988).

We believe that the explanatory models of mental illness (Bentall *et al.*, 1990) can be seen as a shift from those based on extrapolation of invariances (models from the natural sciences) which are either simple reductive etiological or mono-factor or alternatively complex or integrated multi-factor models; to those based on the principle of 'singularisation': the experience or the person as a 'key' for hermeneutic models (e.g. psychodynamic-psychotherapeutic, anthropo-phenomenological).

Using Kuhn's theory, this is a phase of 'revolutionary break' (Kuhn, 1962). De-institutionalisation produced a rupture, a radical change both epistemological and practical. It has modified the course and outcomes of mental disorders becoming preventative from the moment that it intervened in the institution itself, which was the main locus of risk for chronicity, social exclusion, deprivation of power and denial of value to the experiences of the people with those problems (Goffman, 1961; Wing and Brown, 1970; Basaglia, 1987a). We assume here that there is a new model, or a paradigm that derives from de-institutionalisation at its heuristic-operational level. It is based on the principle of complexity through the flexible interaction between observer and observed ('scientists' and 'patients', Maccacaro, 1978). What is pivotal is meaning and sense making within new therapeutic actions, which could be called 'whole life projects' for the people in need (Jenkins and Rix, 2003). We could define it as an 'interactive comprehension model'.

This chapter will demonstrate how de-institutionalisation, from the moment that it problematised the social reintegration of people with mental health problems, can still contribute to produce that change. The present work delineates a number of shifts which are based on practical evidence, as opposed to the evidence-based medicine (Rosen and Teesson, 2001; Rosen *et al.*, 2003). We will also try to explicate certain outcomes, or effects, which can be perceived at the individual level and not just in organisational systems, and attempt to draw some conclusions, which, however, remain absolutely provisional.

Processes: Shifts Based on Practical Evidences

Practice-based Shift One

The passage from psychiatry to mental health can be seen as a movement from total institutions to organisations of human services, featured by programmes, provided by resources, based on relations, which define the pathways of 'demand' for mental health as a 'circuit'.

Closing mental hospitals, particularly in Italy, involved a whole bundle of processes that affect institutional practice and thinking (De Leonardis *et al.*, 1986; Rotelli, 1988). These latter had been built up around the idea of treating the illness; their implications were oppressive, with the loss of rights and power, social exclusion, restraint and violent physical treatments, institutionalism (Wing and Brown, 1970). The re-conversion and re-orientation of economic and human resources, with the mobilisation of all social and institutional actors (workers, patients, families, administrators, laymen), were paralleled by an increase in patients' power and the supply of material support for the discharge and the re-entry into their own community. But in many places institutional practices in health, justice and social service systems still remain.

There is now a new 'circuit' of psychiatric demand, aimed not only at responding but also at control which involves many agencies and services (De Leonardis *et al.*, 1986). The criteria for creating really innovative community services have to be based on the idea that a new organisation in the community must avoid the risks of becoming a new 'diffused' institution, dominated by the idea of only controlling symptoms and behaviours, and discharge/abandonment (Basaglia, 1987a). This is typical of a biological and medicalised psychiatry, which has kept or re-established the distance between professional and patient; it is often done by fragmenting the patient as an 'object' of intervention, as s/he has to fit a service which itself is fragmented into specialised and technical components, hierarchical structures and professional roles. Thus the service is constantly including, excluding and discarding (Dell'Acqua and Mezzina, 1988a, 1988b). The psychiatric system has already defined the narrow band of competencies within which new specialisations can be formed. All such efficiency-based models, founded on a differentiation of facilities, programmes, teams and techniques, provide for the exclusion of 'residuals', which do not fit. These residuals will either never 'come through the door' or will be actively excluded (through selection of demand, or field of intervention) or will be placed in the limited but persistent institutional places of seclusion (De Leonardis *et al.*, 1986).

Hence new solutions of community care can be really effective only if they do not limit themselves as being efficient in terms of the management of target population of service users, defined by their illness features and/or related deviant behaviours (Basaglia, 1987a); but instead must seek to preserve the idea of the person as a whole.

Practice-based Shift Two

A comprehensive service is built up around an holistic view of a person who is supported by 'projects for life'. This continuity of care is in contrast to time limited programmes, whether they be therapeutic or rehabilitative, based upon a 'specialised' array of services, which is often patched and fragmented.

The community service, integrated in its components, has to be seen as the central, unified place/locus, a strategic organisational moment which can direct its vision with the user as central – the active subject – in an agenda of healing, recovery, social restitution and emancipation. We stress here some key-features of that kind, or model, of service (Dell'Acqua and Cogliati Dezza, 1985; De Leonardis *et al.*, 1986; Mosher and Burti, 1989).

Responsibility, Accessibility, Accountability Services which assume full responsibility and commitment to its community, meant as 'catchment area' are actively present. They 'go to meet' the demand and engage in relationships with the individual and groups, the families, housing estates etc. that they encounter. This pro-active approach also helps avoid emergencies, waiting lists, bureaucratic links and referrals and promote an approach of 'shouldering the burden' where people live day to day. Key to this is a full relationship (Mosher and Burti, 1989) with the suffering individual, formed from the onset, from the request for help and aimed at understanding the complexity of the user's situation.

Responding to Comprehensive Needs Interventions, such as those above, progressively reveal the framework of needs, situating the individual once again in an historical-personal perspective within a social network and attribute recognised or visible, personal and interpersonal meaning as mediated amongst the actors who are often involved in conflicting relations. A comprehensive response means firstly enhancing and giving value to the resources present in the user's own living situation, including the contribution of all possible family members (cf. Falloon and Fadden, 1993; Warner, 1985). It comes through a diversification of the Service's own material and human resources, including non-professional and voluntary work, as well as the activation of other services, in order to achieve a wide integration of health and social interventions, therapeutic and supportive. It also creates the concrete possibility of new relationships and new networks of relationships and for changing disruptive repeated patterns in the individual's life.

Social Quality or Community Style Confronting user's needs also means moving the institutional dynamics in a productive direction. Working in teams is fundamental to maximising the Service's human and professional resources. One of the most evident products of de-institutionalisation, and also one of the most powerful factors for change, was the criticism of the rigid, compartmentalised and hierarchical work organisation of the psychiatric hospital (Dell'Acqua and Mezzina, 1988b). The result was a re-negotiation of power amongst the various professional roles, recognizing degrees of responsibility and operational autonomy. The value given to a single worker as a human and technical resource is not the result of service assignments or a mechanical division of labour. It means enhancing each worker's contribution through the assumption of specific tasks and responsibilities within a proper relationship and framed between inter-dependence and operational autonomy. Individuals' autonomy must be constantly verified by the team itself through formal meetings, moments of informal co-operation, the circulation of information and the discussion of projects. This implies a collective 'tension', which works towards consensus within the Service, which establishes effective relationships and also reciprocity. Therefore team work should mean not just a multi-disciplinary approach due to the juxtaposition of professional contributions, but a system of continuous exchanges and the valorisation of every member as a whole person. This is a first step even toward 'recovery' of the professionals themselves (Topor, 2002).

Practice-based Shift Three

From services provided, which are measured by outcomes in term of effectiveness or efficacy, to options/opportunities related to the concept of a personal(sized) 'routes' towards recovery or emancipation.

This implies a different position, active and no longer passive, on the part of the person who suffers. The user is no longer a recipient of care and treatments which is evaluated by the worker in aseptic and spuriously objective terms (as clinical and epidemiological 'outcomes'), but as an actor in his own human itineraries which the Service must facilitate and foster.

The '24 hours community service' signifies a profound change in the operational methods and philosophy of a community service which places the user's life at the very centre of its concerns (Dell'Acqua and Mezzina, 1988a, 1988b; Mosher and Burti, 1989; Reding and Rafelson, 1995; Warner, 1995; Minghella *et al.*, 1998). This is done by using and responding to the 'lived' time, the rhythms and temporal dimension of daily lives, and by catching the interplay between 'health' and 'illness (Basaglia, 1982) as one of its central components.

Continuity of life and continuity of care are therefore linked together. The comprehensive community approach can make the idea of continuity real, both in space and time through the Service/user relationship (Segal, 2004). 'Spatially' in the community means the place for living and where the institutions are located: 'temporally' refers to the periods where there is a need for care, support and rehabilitation. 'Continuity' means following the progress and history of both the individual and the community together. In this way all aspects, prevention, care and rehabilitation will all be dealt with by the Service's practices (De Leonardis *et al.*, 1986).

Assuming a 'position of positive responsibility' is supported by the clear evidence that the 'difficult' demand, in a network of services which operates without psychiatric hospitals, is destined to return, through continuous feedback, to the Service itself, which cannot define the 'end of therapy' in a rigid manner. The Service must be willing to follow the user in a severe condition when he/she drops out and is exposed to sanctions or once again institutional seclusion, such as prisons and forensic hospitals (Dell'Acqua and Mezzina, 1988a, 1988b).

Moreover, the central issue is not only, or no longer, that of simply maintaining the user in his/her social context and fighting exclusion. Therapeutic continuity must be connected to the sense of a 'project for life'. Today's main challenge is the reduction of social harm and the creation of itineraries or networks and pathways for social inclusion as a '(re)production of subjectivity', whilst taking into account the socially disabling impact of experiencing a mental illness (Ciompi, 1984; Harding *et al.*, 1987, 1992; Warner, 1985, 2000). This experience in itself reduces the capacity to access social opportunities, at the same time that they become less affordable because of stigma and discrimination. This leads us to the next point.

Practice-based Shift Four

From formal rights (civil rights), guaranteed by legislation, to social rights linked to the concept of citizenship, and therefore affecting all policies providing resources and bringing about social inclusion.

The priority given to the individual manifests itself in a series of guarantees for his or her full personal realisation, i.e. for the person's full expression as a subject, endowed with power(s). These guarantees should orientate the policies as well as the practices of the Services.

Clearly the WHO campaign 'Stop Exclusion – Dare to Care' (WHO Geneva, 2001) affirmed the importance of rights and users' rights: the right to have one's own living space, regardless of the nature of one's disorder, the right to have an active and productive role in society and the recognition of differences of gender, culture and ethnic origin.

De-institutionalisation has made it possible to re-establish the rights of citizenship for persons affected with mental disorders not only by permitting them to regain a certain level of power, but also by giving them the possibility of having a voice, enabling them to speak, and creating the conditions for the empowerment. It is thus important to understand that alternative practices which are critical of psychiatry are strictly connected to the new forms of self-determination, empowerment and the appearance of users-as-subjects on the social scene, and that there is a link between the possibility of integration and the defense of the value of the experience of suffering as a form of diversity (Mezzina *et al.*, 1992). We underline here that citizenship should be interpreted as a social process that brings about individual and social transformation; thus it is not a status but a 'practice' which is essentially about exercising social rights (De Leonardis, 1997). Hence, it involves a re-distribution of power and a development of capabilities. Moreover, the unresolved tension between specificity (ethnic origin, gender, language) and universality, between diversity and equality, proposes a dialectic node. There is a growing new awareness of the need for culturally-sensitive and culture-bound programmes, whilst not diminishing the struggle for universal access to mainstream services that operate without discrimination and with the maximum flexibility. It means providing wider, more equal access, as against services which discriminate by social class (privatised) and which are profit-based.

Among the actions we can highlight here are networking and the enabling of local community participation in order to ensure 'social mobilisation'. The key to building a community, in the social sense referred to previously, is the building and strengthening of networks. We underline the importance of networks as central to 'creating community' (IMHCN, 2001).

Outcomes: How People Experience the Paradigm Shift

Freedom in mental health means choice, opportunities and alternatives at each phase of the process – from entering to leaving the Service network.

How could this be translated in terms of desirable outcomes directly experienced by people in need?

It obviously implies a range of opportunities to choose (Sen, 1992), ensured by the service in connection with all social and welfare networks. If Services are able to ensure effective and individualised therapeutic/rehabilitative pathways, then choices can be made, counter-proposals discussed and a therapeutic dialogue undertaken with the user.

The de-institutionalisation of the therapeutic relationship is therefore linked to the *recovery* of true 'decision-making' by the user with regards to his/her own life. Regaining power means not only avoiding institutional seclusion or the still existing forms of involuntary treatments and placements, but having a voice, a say through participation and involvement in one's own individual care plan, in the Service itself and in any moment of direct democracy. Thus, we must once again deal with the question of power: workers begin to change when they begin to validate users' subjectivities, and when they can develop a wider alliance against damaging and oppressive routines. All these processes provide the seed for active and collective participation 'through social needs' (e.g. mutual support groups, but also relatives, women and also men addressing issues of gender, young people entering the service network; Mezzina *et al.*, 1992) rather than institutional roles or pathological categories. This leads toward a more advanced and responsible citizens' involvement which regards not only 'primary users' but all people involved in the process and eventually the community (Mezzina *et al.*, 1992).

In this scenario 'recovery' must be linked to notions of emancipation, social inclusion and citizenship, in order to endow the process with more meaning and quality. We must ask ourselves what conception of society and human beings underpins recovery if it is to be regarded as an interpersonal and social fact. If we prefer to speak of recovery and 'emancipation' it is because we wish to underline the lack-of-freedom which is linked to the condition of illness as personal and social misery, the loss of rights, the denial of access to socially exploitable resources; and, conversely, to the effort which must be made in order to 'come back'.

Here it is clear that the Services' role in fostering recovery is through openness, involvement, accessibility and flexibility the possibility of choosing and access to opportunities (Deegan, 1988). Moreover, one of the most important ways out to a social life is provided by the concept of Social Enterprise (Rotelli, 1999). It means creating productive, integrated co-operative societies and social firms that combine different job opportunities and vocational training with user involvement in the economic and decisional structure; but it also means involving the local community and its human and economic resources.

Conclusions

The overall framework of what we sustained here is a parallel movement; from total institutions to community services and from the illness to the person.

This chapter is presenting the cornerstone of a true psychosocial approach, or maybe a true paradigm shift, which is occurring now. The question remains; how can we envisage strategies that do not involve the imposition of power and which enable the person to emerge and grow, making it possible to be a whole person with a whole life in society?

The response still seems to be linked to de-institutionalisation as an important driving force, and its current implications. De-institutionalisation demonstrated how useless and harmful were the institutions of psychiatry. In de-constructing the medical model, attacking the stereotypical, institutional image of illness, de-institutionalisation promoted practical steps in order to abandon the old social exclusion and to promote social re-integration. The main tool is a service, born from those practical evidences, which acts in an integrated way as opposed to the fragmentation of services based on 'reductionist' responses to 'the illness'.

We must envision horizontal organisations, with flat hierarchies, which are internally open and participatory, made up of men and women who work as professional subjects immersed in a community to which they must respond and be accountable. Their practices should be based on the recognition of the user's contribution, either to his/her own or to everybody's mental health. These practices must be accessible to demands and must offer flexible services based on the non-selection of users, maintaining and dealing even with the most difficult conditions within the community. Transformed knowledge, and knowledge which continues to transform itself, comes therefore from practices that 'shoulder the burden', and which actively aid and sustain, step-by-step, the social itinerary of the person who suffers. This synthesis of experience with knowledge frames concepts of practice, which challenge the 'science of psychiatry'. This knowledge, as it circulates and mediates different forms of language, professional knowledge as well as common sense, and moreover the challenge to 'the obvious' (Laing, 1968), involves many players through sharing the power, and becomes the tool for bringing about change. We believe that a transformed subjectivity is produced in a relationship which breaks the rules (Topor, 2002) by permitting both the worker and the user to express themselves, thereby enabling another actor – the community – to enter. In a certain sense, therapeutic practice must go beyond itself; it must promote 'life' in order to produce 'health'. In a de-institutionalised model we consider illness as an event which is constructed at that point where the personal, subjective, social and institutional interlock and intersect (Maccacaro, 1978). It can be thereby deconstructed, disassembling the illness as 'suffering' – an event in the person's life journey which comes into contact with the institutional agent, the Service. If at the centre of psychiatric practices is the search for, and production of meaning (Weick, 1995) as well as recovery processes, the problem of a 'return to the community' for each person who has travelled the road of loneliness and pain can be successfully universalised.

References

Andrews, G., Teesson, M., Stewart, G. and Hoult, J. (1990), 'Follow-up of community placement of the chronic mentally ill in New South Wales', *Hospital and Community Psychiatry*, 41 (2) 184-188.

Basaglia, F. (1987), 'Institutions of Violence', in Nancy Scheper Hughes and Anne Lowell (eds), *Psychiatry Inside-out: Selected Writings of Franco Basaglia*, New York: Columbia University Press.

Basaglia, F. (1987a), 'The disease and its double and the deviant majority', in Nancy Scheper Hughes and Anne Lowell (eds), *Psychiatry Inside-out. Selected Writings of Franco Basaglia*, New York: Columbia University Press.

Basaglia, F. (1987b), 'Letter from America: The artificial patient', in Nancy Scheper Hughes and Anne Lowell (eds), *Psychiatry Inside-out. Selected Writings of Franco Basaglia*. New York: Columbia University Press.

Basaglia, F. (1987c), 'Madness/Delirium', in Nancy Scheper Hughes and Anne Lowell (eds), *Psychiatry Inside-out. Selected Writings of Franco Basaglia*, New York: Columbia University Press.

Basaglia, F. (1982), 'Il concetto di salute e malattia', F. Basaglia, *Scritti* (ed.), Vol. II, Torino: Einaudi.

Bauman, Z. (2000), *Liquid Modernity*, Oxford: Polity Press: Cambridge and Blackwell Publishers Ltd.

Bentall. R. (ed.) (1990), *Reconstructing Schizophrenia*, London: Routledge.

Castel, R. (1976*), L'Ordre Psychiatrique. L'Age d'Or de l'Aliénisme*, Paris: Les Editions De Minuits.

Castel, R. (1982,), 'La società psichiatrica avanzata', *Aut-Aut*, 182.

Ciompi, L. (1983), 'How to improve the treatment of schizophrenics: A multicausal illness concept and its therapeutic consequences', in Sterlin, H., Wynne, C. and Wirsching, M. (eds), *Social Intervention in Schizophrenia*, Berlin: Springer.

Ciompi, L. (1984), 'Is there a schizophrenia? The Long Term Course of Psychotic Phenomena', *British Journal of Psychiatry*, **145**: 636-640.

Ciompi, L., Dauwalder, H.P., Maier, C., Aebi, E., Truetsch, K., Kupper, Z. and Rutishauser, C. (1992), 'The Pilot-Project "Soteria Berne". Clinical experiences and results', *British Journal of Psychiatry*, 161: 145-153.

Crow, T. and Deakin, B. (eds) (1987), *Transmission: Biological Psychiatry in Clinical Practice*, London: Education in Practice.

Dean, C., Phillips, J., Gadd, E., Joseph, M. and England, S. (1993), 'Comparison of a community-based service with a hospital-based service for people with acute, severe psychiatric illness', *British Medical Journal*, 307: 473-476.

Deegan, P.E. (1988), 'Recovery: The lived experience of rehabilitation', *Psychosocial Rehabilitation Journal*, 11(4), 11-19.

De Leonardis, O. (1997), *Il Terzo Escluso*, Milano: Feltrinelli.

De Leonardis, O., Mauri, D. and Rotelli, F. (1986), 'Deinstitutionalization: A different path. The Italian Mental Health Reform', *Health Promotion*, W.H.O: Cambridge University Press 2, 151-165.

Deleuze, G. and Guattari, F. (1972), *L'Anti-Oedipe*, Paris: Les Editions Des Minuit.

Dell'Acqua, G. and Cogliati Dezza, M.G. (1985), 'The end of the mental hospital: A review of the psychiatric experience in Trieste', *Acta Psychiatrica Scandinavica*, Supplement. 316, 45-69.

Dell'Acqua, G. and Mezzina, R. (1988a), 'Approaching Mental Distress', in Ramon, S. and Giannichedda, M.G. (eds), *Psychiatry in Transition: The British and Italian Experiences.* London: Pluto Press.

Dell'Acqua, G. and Mezzina, R. (1988b), 'Responding to crisis: Strategies and intentionality in community psychiatric intervention', Per *La Salute Mentale/For Mental Health*, 1 Centro Studi Salute Mentale: Trieste.

Falloon, I.R.H. and Fadden, G. (1993), *Integrated Mental Health Care: A Comprehensive Community Based Approach*, New York: Cambridge University Press.

Fenton, W.S., Mosher, L.R., Herrell, J.M. and Blyler, C.R. (1998), 'Randomized trial of general hospital and residential alternative care for patients with severe and persistent mental illness', *American Journal of Psychiatry*, 155: 516-522.

Foucault, M. (1972), *L'historie de la Folie à l'Age Classique*, Paris: Gallimard.

Goffman, E. (1961), *Asylums. Essays on the Social Situation of Mental Patients and Other Inmate*, New York: Anchor Books, Doubleday & Co.

Harding, C.M., Zubin, J. and Strauss, J.S. (1987), 'Chronicity in schizophrenia: Fact, partial act or artifact?', *Hospital and Community Psychiatry*, 38, 477-486.

Harding, C.M., Zubin, J. and Strauss, J.S. (1992), 'Chronicity in schizophrenia: Revisited'. *British Journal of Psychiatry*, 161, 27-37.

Hoult, J. and Reynolds, I. (1984), 'Schizophrenia: A comparative trial of community oriented and hospital oriented psychiatric care', *Acta Psychiatrica Scandinavica*, 69: 359-372.

Hoult, J., Rosen, A. and Reynolds I. (1984), 'Community orientated treatment compared to psychiatric hospital orientated treatment', *Social Science and Medicine*, 11: 1005-1010.

Hoult, J. (1986), 'The community care of the acutely mentally ill', *British Journal of Psychiatry*, 149: 137-144.

Husserl, E. (1970), *The Crisis of European Science and Transcendental Phenomenology*, Evanston, Il: Northwestern University Press.

International Mental Health Collaborative Network (2001), 'Foundation Document', www.imhcn.com.

Jones, M. (1974), *Beyond the Therapeutic Community. Social Learning and Social Psychiatry*, Yale University Press: Yale.

Jenkins, J. and Rix, S. (2003), 'The Whole Life Programme'. National Institute Mental Health Excellence: East Region.

Kuhn, T. (1962), *The Structure of Scientific Revolutions*, Chicago: University of Chicago Press.

Laing, R.D. (1968), 'The Obvious', in Cooper, D. (ed.), *The Dialectics Of Liberation*, Penguin Books: Harmondsworth.

Maccacaro, G.A. (1978), 'Appunti per una ricerca su: epidemiologia dell'istituzione psichiatrica come malattia sociale', *Fogli d'informazione*, 50: 306-310.

Marks, I.M., Connolly, J., Muijen, M. and Audini, B. (1994), 'Home based versus hospital based care for people with severe mental illness', *British Journal of Psychiatry*, 165: 179-194.

Mezzina, R., Mazzuia, M., Vidoni, D. and Impagnatiello, M. (1992), 'Networking consumers participation in a community mental health service: Mutual support groups, citizenship, coping strategies', *International Journal of Social Psychiatry*, 38 (1), 68-73.

Mezzina, R. and Vidoni, D. (1995), 'Beyond the mental hospital: Crisis and continuity of care in Trieste. A four-year follow-up study in a community mental health centre', *The International Journal of Social Psychiatry*, 41: 1-20.

Minghella, E., Ford, R., Freeman, T., Hoult, J., McGlynn, P.E. and O'Halloran, P. (1998), *Open All Hours. 24-Hour Response for People with Mental Health Emergencies*, London: The Sainsbury Centre For Mental Health.

Moltzen, S., Gurevitz, H., Rappaport, M. and Goldman H.H. (1986), 'The psychiatric health facility: An alternative of acute inpatient treatment in a non hospital setting', *Hospital and Community Psychiatry*, 37: 1131-35.

Mosher, L.R. and Burti, L. (1989), *Community Mental Health. Principles and Practice*, London: W.W. Norton & Co.

Mosher, L.R. and Menn, A.Z. (1977), 'Lowered barriers in the community: The Soteria Model', in Stein, L.A. and Test, M.A. (eds), *Alternatives To Mental Hospital Treatment*, New York: Plenum Press.

Mosher, L.R. and Menn, A.Z. (1989), 'Community residential treatment: Alternatives to hospitalization', in A. Bellack (ed.), *A Clinical Guide For The Treatment Of Schizophrenia*, New York: Plenum Press.

Polak, P.R. and Kirby, M.W. (1976), 'A model to replace psychiatric hospitals', *The Journal of Nervous And Mental Disease*, 13-22.

Porter, R. (1987), *A Social History of Madness. The World Through The Eyes of The Insane*, Grove/Atlantic.

Reding, G.R. and Raphelson, M. (1995), 'Around the clock mobile psychiatric crisis intervention: Another effective alternative to psychiatric hospitalisation', *Community Mental Health Journal* 31: 179-187.

Rosen, A., Diamond, R.J., Miller, V. and Stein, L.I. (1997), 'Becoming real: From model programs to implemented services', in E.J. Hollingsworth (ed.), *The Successful Diffusion of Innovative Program Approaches. New Directions for Mental Health Services, No. 74.* San Francisco: Jossey-Bass.

Rosen, A. and Teesson, M. (2001), 'Does case management work? The evidence and the abuse of evidence-based medicine', *Australian And New Zealand Journal of Psychiatry*, **35**: 731-746.

Rosen, A., Newton, L. and Barfoot, K. (2003), 'Evidence based community alternatives to institutional psychiatric care', *Medicine Today*, **4** (9), 90-95.

Rotelli, F. (1988), 'Changing Psychiatric Services in Italy', in Ramon, S. and Giannichedda, M.G. (eds), *Psychiatry in Transition: The British and Italian Experiences*, London: Pluto Press.

Rotelli, F. (1999), 'Per Un'Impresa Sociale', in F. Rotelli, *Per la normalità – taccuino di uno psichiatra negli anni della Grande Riforma*, Seconda Edizione, Asterios, Trieste.

Sartre, J.P. (1960), *Critique de la Raison Dialectique*, Gallimard: Paris.

Segal, S.P. (2004), 'Taking issue: Managing transitions and ensuring good care', *Psychiatric Services*, 55, November, 1205.

Sen, A. (1992), *Inequality Reexamined*, Oxford: Oxford University Press.

Smyth, M.G. and Hoult, J. (2000), 'The home treatment enigma', *British Medical Journal*, 320 (7230): 305-308.

Stein, L.I. and Test, M.A. (1978), 'An alternative to mental hospital treatment, in Stein, L.A. and Test, M.A. (eds), *Alternatives to Mental Hospital Treatment*, New York: Plenum Press.

Stein, L.I. and Test, M.A. (eds) (1985), *Training in the Community Living Model – A Decade of Experience. New Directions for Mental Health Services, 26*, San Francisco: Jossey-Bass.

Strauss, J.S. and Carpenter, W.T. (1981), *Schizophrenia*, Plenum: New York.

Topor, A. (2002), *Managing the Contradictions. Recovery from Severe Mental Disorders.* Stockholm: Stockholm University, Department of Social Work.

Tosquelles, F. (1992), *L'Enseignement de la Folie*, Toulouse: Éditions Privat.

Warner, R. (1985), *Recovery from Schizophrenia. Psychiatry and Political Economy*, London: Routledge and Kegan Paul.

Warner, R. (2000), *The Environment of Schizophrenia. Innovation In Practice, Policy And Communications*, London: Brunner-Routledge.

Warner, R. (ed.) (1995), *Alternatives to Hospital for Acute Psychiatric Treatment*, Washington, DC: American Psychiatry Press.

Weick K.E. (1995), *Sensemaking in Organizations*, Sage: London.

Wing, J.K. and Brown, G.W. (1970), *Institutionalism and Schizophrenia*, Cambridge, MA: Cambridge University Press.

World Health Organization (1986), 'Declaration of Human Rights', Ottawa: WHO.

World Health Organization (2001), 'Stop exclusion – Dare to care. World Health Day 2001', Department of Mental Health and Substance Abuse: Geneva, WHO/NMH/MSD/WHD/00.2.

Zubin, J. and Spring, B. (1977), 'Vulnerability – a new view of schizophrenia', *Journal of Abnormal Psychology*, 86(2) 103-126.

Chapter 7

Structural Issues Underpinning Mental Health Care and Psychosocial Approaches in Developing Countries: The Brazilian Case

Eduardo Mourão Vasconcelos

1. Introduction

This chapter aims at providing:

- a framework for analyzing mental health care and psychosocial approaches in Third World countries, from a cross-national comparative perspective.
- an overview of this sector in Brazil, from both historical and descriptive perspectives, illustrating the current direction of implementing the psychiatric reform, its internal and external dynamics, using the analytical framework outlined in the first section.
- a review of the main practical and political strategies used in the development of psychosocial rehabilitation approaches in Brazil, as an example of the typical challenges in the present wider context of Third World countries of structural adjustment, fiscal crisis of the state, increasing poverty, unemployment and social violence.

2. Cross-national Comparative Framework for Analyzing the Historical Dynamics of Mental Health Systems and Psychosocial Rehabilitation Programmes

A critical understanding the dynamics of mental health systems and psychosocial perspectives in developing countries requires a wider comparative approach, mainly from the perspective of those living in central highly developed nations. Classical studies have shown that Third World countries witness very complex patterns of 'unequal and combined' economic, political, social and cultural development (Oliveira, 1976; Velho, 1976; Da Matta, 1979). For this purpose, an analytical framework developed by the author will be proposed below (Vasconcelos, 1992).

Political contexts of democratization, revolutionary waves and reaffirmation of civil and political rights, tend to stimulate the acknowledgement of the rights of people with mental illness, particularly those still living in asylums or using in-patient settings. In particular, the organization of networks of mutual support and the political mobilization of mental health workers, users, their relatives and allied social movements have been a key element for initiating the process of psychiatric reform and the development of critical psychosocial approaches. Unlike most developed nations, Third World countries tend to show a much more unstable political scenario, with mental health systems and the development of psychosocial programmes highly dependent on such changes and on the direct political action taken by stakeholders in the field.

The existence of strong networks of informal social care, particularly extended families, neighbourhoods, religious and ethnic communities, have been a crucial element in ensuring long term good outcome from severe mental health illnesses (Ciompi, 1980; Davidson and McGlashan, 1997; Lin and Kleinman, 1988; McGlashan, 1988). From a parallel perspective, demographic changes, particularly the increase of the elderly in the general population and changes in the family structure, may lead to the development of social services which substitute family informal care. Therefore, Third World countries with predominant hierarchical cultural systems and still in early stages of the demographic transition tend to present better prospects for recovery in the mental health field than developed nations, particularly those with a highly individualistic culture and in late stages of the demographic transition, even with the development of welfare systems.

The development of welfare systems and emphasis on social rights is a key element allowing the implementation of community mental health services along the network of other community care settings and personal social services. Social insurance schemes for disabled people guarantees a minimum income, which allows the provision of care in the community, even in the absence of employment opportunities. Equally, the development of public health ideas and the implementation of health systems politically committed to universal and high standard of care provides a favourable environment for the provision of integrated out-patient mental health services. Furthermore, psychosocial approaches depend significantly on the internal inter-institutional flexibility of the welfare system in integrating different funding lines and branches of insurance, health, mental health and social services. Third World countries tend to show very poor, non-universal, non-flexible and unequal welfare and health systems, compensated by the traditional strong provision of informal care. However, transitional patterns, particularly in large urban environments, may present a real challenge for the development of good mental health care in the community. Similarly, the present hegemony of neo-liberal adjustment policies and of crisis of welfare systems, even in developed countries, has led to de-hospitalization policies without the parallel provision of enough or good quality out-patient care, provoking serious setbacks in the already established network of community services. However, this challenge is particularly amplified in Third World nations, subjected to unequal international relations and to enormous pressure to pay their external debt, where committed de-institutionalization policies require fine balancing in establishing the right pace for advancing the process without creating more social negligence.

Economic contexts of shortage of labour and revaluing human labour stimulates the investment in effective rehabilitation of population groups hitherto considered unproductive, including the mentally ill (Warner, 1985). From the opposite perspective, historical contexts of unemployment and loss of labour rights make it more difficult for dependent social groups to find employment and socially valued activities, decreasing the general revenue for funding social policies in general, and leading to deterioration in the working conditions of mental health workers. Third World countries present a large tertiary service sector, with wider possibilities for informal activities. However, the present context of structural unemployment across the capitalist world has posed real challenges to the development of occupational schemes, a crucial element of psychosocial rehabilitation. Moreover, the deterioration in employment conditions is undermining the commitment of mental health workers to the intrinsic challenges of community care.

Historical contexts of war and natural catastrophes reinforce national solidarity and stimulate the rehabilitation of soldiers and civilians with post-traumatic distresses, in a process similar to shortage of labour. The development of therapeutic communities during World War II in the UK is a good example of this, triggering the gradual acknowledgement of how a participative environment with a wide range of social and cultural opportunities is a key element for recovery and psychosocial approaches.

The historical features of professionalism in the mental health field, particularly medicine and psychiatry, psychology, social work and nursing, represent a central element in the development of mental health community care and psychosocial approaches. Professionalism includes specific patterns in the historical development of the technical and social division of labour, the acknowledgement of mastery over specific fields of knowledge and practice, the establishment of corporative organizations, and specific professional cultures (Ramon, 1987; Vasconcelos, 2002). The varied social mandates and professional cultures imply different scientific paradigms, theories, expertise and practices, as well as culturally rooted conceptualizations of mental phenomena, co-existing with very rigid boundaries among them. From the opposite perspective, community care and psychosocial approaches are very sensitive to frameworks able to recover the complexity and multidimensionality of human reality, as well as to the possibility of interdisciplinary conceptualization and professional practice (Vasconcelos, 2002).

The development and diffusion of new therapeutic ideas and practices, particularly from the twentieth century, in psychology (psychoanalysis, phenomenology, analytical psychology) and pharmacology (the new psycho-active drugs from the late fifties onwards) has been a stimulating element in the implementation of community care. In-depth approaches have allowed understanding the unconscious and the odd aspects of mental illness, showing that similar psychological processes are present in every human being, breaking the hitherto sharp distinction between normal and abnormal states. Overall, the twentieth century's new therapeutic practices have not only rejected the removal of the distressed individual from the ordinary environment, but also helped to understand and control the more disruptive symptoms for both acute and chronic users in the community (Busfield, 1986; Warner, 1985; Scull, 1984).

3. The Reform of the Brazilian Mental Health System: A Historical Perspective

Brazil is viewed as a Third World nation, due to the following:

Although rated as the 15th economy on the planet in 2003 (O Globo, 01/10/2003: 21), the country's division of labour and of financial flows are those of a typical Third World nation, with main exports in the agriculture sector and huge external debt, around 56 per cent of the GNP, obliging the government to divert most of the internal revenue to paying the debt service;

Its social profile is also similar to Third World nations. Brazil has been classified as having one of the worst social inequality profile in the world. In the year 2000, the richest 10 per cent of the population had an income 46 times bigger than the poorest 10 per cent, in a process that has been accelerated in the last 40 years (O Globo, 30/09/2003: 19). The international scale for Human Development Rate located Brazil in the 79th place (PNUD, 1999, in Enciclopedia do Mundo Contemporâneo, 2000: 79), after countries such as the Philippines, Lebanon, Libya, Colombia, Suriname and Russia. Infantile mortality is also very high, being classified also in the 79th place in 1998 (UNICEF, 1998, in op cit: 72), with a higher rate than Botswana, Vietnam, El Salvador and other known Third World nations. Therefore, although presenting some features of a developed country, particularly for the rich, a large part of the population presents a social profile very similar to Third World nations.

Thus far from the relatively stable picture of highly developed countries, the dynamics of the mental health system in Third World nations is strongly dependent on the larger political, economic and social scenario, with deep changes within short periods of time.

Stages in the Development of the Psychiatric Reform in Brazil

The psychiatric reform in Brazil has been carried out now for at least 26 years, beginning during its military dictatorship in 1978. At this time, like other Latin American countries, the Brazilian population has witnessed between 1964 and 1984 one of the darkest periods of its history, due to a dictatorship that controlled coercively all political, social and cultural life.

The stages of the reform include:

The first period (1978–1992) was marked by open denounces and mobilization of public opinion against a psychiatric care only based on large and closed psychiatric institutions, by a social movement composed only by mental health workers. The mental health movement has had strong links to others social movements that, from 1978 onwards, have also emerged from the underground activities during the darkest years of the dictatorship. Among them, it is important to remember the 'Sanitário Movement' (Public health movement), a strong alliance that started up a profound change in the public health sector, towards the creation of an universal national health system, also inspired in the British NHS.

The second period (1982–1992), that began still under military rule at national level, but with its end in 1984, witnessed a larger process of political re-democratization. In the mental health sector, it was marked by the entry of health and mental health movement leaders (still formed only by mental health workers) to the state institutions, after elections and victory of democratic forces at some of the main states of the federation, pushing ahead statutory mental health programmes, in parallel with the creation of a national health system, towards:

- controlling administratively and clinically the access to in-patient care
- implementing first programmes designed to 'humanize' these institutional settings
- attempting to set up out-patient clinics and multiprofessional teams mainly inspired by French 'sector psychiatry' and North American 'preventative psychiatry'
- consolidating the achievements of the struggle against the dictatorship, with a new Constitution in 1988, that also established the guidelines for a new universal public health system
- reaching out a consensus on the reform's agenda, through the organization of the first National Mental Health Conference, in 1987
- still during this period, a more radical branch of the mental health movement has emerged in 1987, called 'Anti-manicomial Movement' ('against the madhouse'), against all forms of specialized in-patient care, inspired by the Italian experience, setting out gradually the political orientation which would be hegemonic during the next period.

The third period (1992–1996) has been marked by a first wave of institutionalization of the National Health System ('Sistema Único de Saúde', or shortly, SUS) and of a clear but gradual psychiatric de-institutionalization strategy, inspired by the Italian Democratic Psychiatry model, looking at:

- implementing the National Health System, established by the new democratic Federal Constitution of 1988 and by specific legislation issued in 1990. Its conceptualization is inspired on World Health Organization's ideas, particularly on the Alma Ata International Conference (UNICEF, 1978), and based on principles like universalisation, regionalisation, descentralisation and participation (Carvalho and Santos, 1992; Fleury, 1997)
- organizing the 2nd National Mental Health Conference in 1992, after a two-year process of meetings and conferences at local, regional and each state levels, which established a strong consensus towards the new strategy in the field

- consolidating a larger and grass-rooted Anti-manicomial Movement, pushing ahead the claims for de-institutionalized care in the community, with local, regional and national militant collectives and meetings
- supporting the organization of the first user and relatives' groups and associations, although still assisted and supported by mental health workers and services, with increasing presence of their leaders and representatives in events and policy councils in the mental health field, at city, state and national levels
- setting up financial provision for and implementing psychosocial rehabilitation services in the community, with parallel gradual decrease in the number of conventional psychiatric beds (a description of mental health services will be outlined below)
- maintaining a long process of parliamentary debate over new psychiatric legislation at national, state and local authority levels
- creating and diffusing events and post-graduation programmes for training professionals to work and to develop research through the new policy perspective.

The fourth period can be identified between *1996 and 2000*, marked by a temporary stagnation in the advancement of initiatives and policies at national level and slower consolidation at local and state levels, due to the following constraints:

- The federal government, led by the social democrat sociologist Fernando Henrique Cardoso, has implemented a clear neo-liberal programme, undermining statutory policies in the social and health fields, increasing unemployment, social inequality, exclusion, poverty, violence and diffusing an insensitive managerial culture in the statutory administration
- Specifically in the health and mental health sectors, the federal government opted out for a conservative leadership and agenda, freezing temporarily the efforts for the consolidation of the SUS (National Health System) and of the psychiatric reform
- There has been a strong re-organization of the conventional lines of psychiatric research and practice, reinforced by recent neuro-chemical, genetic and technological developments.

The fifth period started up in *2000*. There has been no significant change in the wider political, economic, social policy and general social context, marked by increasing poverty and violence, even with the new federal government by the leftist Worker's Party, which came to power in January 2003. Nevertheless, there has been an assertive political action by the Anti-manicomial and Psychiatric Reform social movements, towards occupying the new political space within the administration at national and each state and local authority levels, particularly opened by Ministries of Health more committed with the SUS during the period, achieving a new wave of administrative, legislative and service initiatives, such as:

- approving a new Psychiatric Law (April 2001), consolidating the reform agenda and several user rights, issuing new administrative and financial provisions enabling diverting funds from in-patient to out-patient care, controlling quality of care in in-patient settings, funding new residential services and reshaping and increasing the number of open mental health centres in the community
- organizing the 3rd National Mental Health Conference in 2001, after several meetings and conferences at all levels of the country, having up-dated and reinforced the political consensus on the continuation of the reform's values and process
- implementing the first experiences of integrating mental health services and the recently established network of health promotion community teams (mainly the so-called Family Health Programme – PSF), with small groups of doctors, nurses and staff visiting and caring for people at their own houses, within a larger reference and counter-reference system for more complex cases
- broadening the scope of policy, care and services to integrate new issues and clientele groups under the de-institutionalization strategy, taking the first initiatives towards drug abuse, child and teenage, elderly, forensic psychiatry, and HIV positive groups
- increasing the number of user and family associations in all the country, generally mixed with some committed professionals, with a parallel diffusion of empowerment approaches, particularly systematized by the present paper's author (Vasconcelos, 1999, 2000, 2002, 2003). This process has led to a division in the original Anti-manicomial movement, mainly between those militant professionals who emphasize direct political action within state apparatuses as against mental health workers, users and family leaders who focused more on the importance of local and grass-root empowerment strategies
- despite all these developments specific to the mental health field, the systematic adherence to neo-liberal structural adjustment policies at national level has led to a continued economic and social decline, in parallel with a significant increase in the rate of unemployment, low wages, poverty, social inequality and violence. This picture has consistently undermined the efforts to reform mental health services in a larger scale and in a quicker pace. It has made it much more difficult for users and families to find jobs, social opportunities and housing in the community. In addition, the spread of drug dealing and consumption has provoked a sharp increase in urban violence and in the number of those requiring mental health care. Larger areas of the open urban space in big cities tend to be considered now as unhealthy and dangerous, requiring residents to keep to their houses or to closed collective spaces like shopping centres, particularly for people with any kind of disability. In such an environment, the sense of reaching out in the community and community action is significantly weakened and de-stimulated
- since 1977, during almost three decades of psychiatric reform, the long-term demographic and cultural changes in the country has sharply decreased the

ability for family and community informal care provision, particularly in larger cities. These changes include, for example, a higher proportion of the elderly in the general population; the disorganization of the traditional nuclear or extended family, with a huge decrease in the average number of children per family and a major increase in the number of single households and of homelessness. This context deserves particular concern when considering the inability of the Brazilian welfare system to respond adequately to the new level of personal social care needs, given the crisis of all statutory policies and the inadequacy of neo-liberal macro-economic policies to offer new solutions.

4. Strategies for Change: Current Mental Health Services and Challenges

The current service profile will be outlined below, through the description of the main strategies adopted to carry on the process of psychiatric reform.

A rigid control over quality of life and care inside all in-patient settings, triggering the process of closure of hospitals

During the two periods of greater political mobilization in the field (1992–1996, 2000–2004), the main strategy for de-hospitalization has been the establishment of special evaluation committees in each state to scrutinize the quality of care inside conventional psychiatric hospitals. Their aim was to promote humanization and quality of care, and to propose special intervention committees for facilities with lower standards, thus generating a gradual process of closure, which included an individualized assessment of each in-patient, preparation for resettlement the establishment of a service network in the community.

The changes in the number of beds in psychiatric hospitals in all the country, during the last 13 years, is shown in Table 7.1.

Table 7.1   Number of beds in psychiatric hospitals over time

Year	1991	1996	1999	2001	2003/2004
Number of beds	82,549	72,970	61,393	54,141	52,406

Sources: Alves, 1992; Delgado *et al.*, 2001; Ministério da Saúde – Coordenação Geral de saúde Mental, 2003–2004.

The Ministry of Health's General Coordination for Mental Health estimates that the present total of conventional psychiatric beds in the country (52,406 in 2003/2004, for a total population of 170 million inhabitants in 2000), still utilises around 85 per cent of the financial provision in the mental health field, as compared to 95 per cent of all provisions in 1990. Around 40,000 of those beds are for long stay in-patients. A high proportion of the total amount of beds are located in large institutions with more than 400 beds, mainly in larger cities, with a significant number of residents with more than a year of stay. It is possible to estimate that a third of the in-patients cannot leave the hospital only due to lack of family and social care in the community. The main reasons for such a slow process has been:

- the in-population profile, most of them very old, highly dependent on intensive care, and without any family ties in the community
- the political, financial and administrative difficulties in establishing residential services and providing direct grants to users in the process of discharge.

Establishing Residential Services and Direct Grants for Users/Families in Process of Resettlement

Several attempts to provide funding for housing during the 1990s have been blocked for political and administrative reasons, resistance from the traditional psychiatric hospital sector and difficulties in allowing public health funds to pay for services considered essentially as providing social, rather than health, care. These obstacles had been overcome only in 2000, when a specific provision has been finally approved. In 2004, there are 189 statutory residential services in all the country, housing 1009 people. An additional provision was issued in 2003 to supply direct grants to users and/or their families, with only 206 people receiving them by February 2004.

Implementing a Network of Psychosocial Care Centres ('Centros de Atenção Psicossocial', or CAPS)

During the process of psychiatric reform, three main types of CAPS have been developed:

- a very informal day centre, with a small interdisciplinary team providing ad hoc workshops, socio-cultural and sports activities
- a formal day centre, with a large range of activities from 8:00 AM to 6:00 PM, staffed with 10/20-member interdisciplinary teams
- a systematic 24-hour-a-day centre, open 7 days a weak, with some beds for crisis intensive care, inspired by the Italian Trieste model, acknowledged as able to substitute in full the conventional in-patient care.

Most centres existing in Brazil represent the two first models, as the third one requires a large amount of funding, staffing, political will and strong commitment by mental health workers. Their diffusion within the country is very uneven, concentrated in larger and medium size cities mainly in South-East states, the more populous and rich. Catchment areas size may present sharp variations, from 70,000 (the ideal proposed by the National Coordination) to more than 1 million inhabitants, and most services have nowadays their caseload full.

Practically all CAPS-type services in the country are provided directly by the statutory sector, or contracted out by the former to the voluntary sector. Conventional psychiatry/psychology and their private-for-profit services have demonstrated no interest at all in the development of such kind of care, considered labour intensive, expensive and too complex, in relation to their traditional specialized practices.

The evolution in the number of CAPS during the last few years in all the country is shown in Table 7.2.

Table 7.2   Number of Psychosocial Care Centres (CAPS) over time

Year	1997	1999	2001	2003/2004
Number of CAPS	176	237	266	500

Sources: Delgado *et al.*, 2001; Ministério da Saúde – Coordenação Geral de saúde Mental, 2003–2004.

There is substantive evidence to demonstrate that the major part of the present network of CAPS can play a central pole in their catchment areas, and is effective in decreasing substantially or even in avoiding new admissions for those in care. However, a network based only on day centres is still fragile to function as the main basis for acute care, still located in conventional emergency services. It is also insufficient in looking after those discharged from long stay wards in conventional asylums, normally requiring residential settings with more intensive, continuous, care.

The CAPS' daily activities vary largely with the clientele and with the socio-economic, cultural and clinical features of the area. Arts, sports, music, dance, physical, educational and occupational workshops, group dynamics and meetings, represent the most common profile. Due to high rates of unemployment (a reliable research organization funded by the trade union movement in the country – DIEESE – has estimated that unemployment in 2004 has reached 20 per cent of the active population), and in response to the diffuse urban violence, the low level of social care provided by the country's welfare state, users stick to their CAPS and reject reaching out initiatives. This context has led to a kind of 'cronification' of the clientele, similar to that observed in conventional psychiatric hospitals and to the bureaucratization of conventional out-patient services. The most recent strategies attempting to change this are: (1) transforming day-centres into 24-hour centres, more centred on those needing acute care, change that will take a slow pace, due to funding constraints; (2) refer those more advanced in their recovery process to the redesigned integrated and flexible out-patient consultation services, particularly in highly populated urban areas; (3) stimulate empowerment initiatives, particularly mutual support occupational and housing projects.

The Integration of Psychosocial Care Centres within the Health Promotion Teams' Network

As indicated in the historical outline above, since the early 1990s there has been in Brazil a consistent policy towards implementing health promotion programmes

(Family Health Programme – 'Programa de Saúde da Família', PSF and Community Health Agents Programme – 'Programa de Agentes Comunitários de Saúde', PACS), particularly in poorest country and rural areas (Souza, 2001a, 2001b, 2002; Pinheiro and Mattos, 2001).

The implementing team consists of a doctor, a nurse, an auxiliary nurse, and between four to six trained local residents, though other professionals such as psychologists and social workers may be added to the team or may be included in background support teams. The latter represents the most common strategy in the mental health field, particularly through mobilizing regular professionals of the nearest CAPS, which are responsible for training the local area teams and represents the reference service for more complex cases. Each team has a caseload of 2,400 to 4,500 people, who should be visited regularly at their own houses. Around one third of the general population in the country, almost 60 millions inhabitants, have been covered now by such teams.

The programme offers a series of priority duties, including nutrition, care for the newborns and their mothers, vaccination, health education and sanitation. Other issues have been also included in several experiences within the country, including direct mental health interventions. From a comparative perspective with developed countries, the health promotion programme in Brazil has worked as the first systematic pattern of community care or personal social services. Only gradually have other initiatives been launched more recently focusing larger social issues, also centred on families. This process is understandable, as the public health social movement in Brazil advanced these kind of initiatives since the late seventies and is much stronger than the other stakeholders in the social field, and therefore it functions as the vanguard of all types of social care in the community. On the other hand, in such a context of lack of a larger network of social care, health promotion teams normally find very complex and difficult situations and challenges in their daily work, without actual resources to deal properly with them. This adds up a lot of stress and burden on health workers'.

The Promotion of Participation, Accountability and Empowerment

The Brazilian Public Health System's (Sistema Único de Saúde – SUS) organization is planned to promote participation and a decision sharing process that includes users, relatives and consumers. Decision making councils should have the last word in every catchment area and at municipality, state and federal levels. In addition, general policy guidelines are discussed in large conferences at each level, which chooses representatives to national conferences, considered the main forum for decisions. Half of the seats at each council and in the local, regional or national conferences, are taken by users or civil society's representatives. There have been specific conferences on general public health, epidemiological vigilance and on mental health.

In practice, most of the social policy councils have been politically and administratively manipulated by city mayors and policy managers. However, where stakeholders are politically active, particularly in the public health and the Anti-manicomial social movements, health councils can be very participative and responsible for the main decisions. Equally, the strategy designed for setting national policy agenda on national conferences, preceded by local and regional conferences, has demonstrated a very high level of commitment and participation since the early 1990s.

Empowerment is also stimulated in the mental health field through the creation of users and family associations at service or local level, generally with the support of more engaged professionals. However, as a more recent trend, there is no reliable data on the exact number of such groups and associations in the country. Nevertheless, user and family leaders have usually been invited to speak up in most of the public events in the field throughout the country.

Summary

From the perspective of those living in highly developed capitalist countries, the transcultural experience of making sense of the reality in Third World nations represents usually a very difficult task. A complex pattern of economic, social, cultural and social policy development has been demonstrated as typical to the Brazilian context. I hope that this chapter will help readers to accomplish an understanding of the main features of our mental health field, by proposing a set of structural parameters for comparative analysis. The historical and descriptive outline provided would enable readers to assess the sensitivity necessary in implementing de-institutionalization policies and psychosocial programmes in such an unfavorable economic, political and social context present nowadays in countries like ours.

Above all, however, it is my wish that this chapter should stimulate and invite further contact with our country and our culture. From this perspective, despite all challenges and oddities, Brazilians are widely known for their friendship, cheerfulness and hospitality.

References

Alves, D.S. (1992), 'Transformações da assistência psiquiátrica no Brasil', in J. Russo e J.F. Silva Filho, *Duzentos anos de psiquiatria*, Rio de Janeiro, UFRJ/Relume Dumará.

Busfield, J. (1986), *Managing madness: Changing ideas and practices*, London, Hutchinson.

Carvalho, G.I. e Santos, L. (1992), *Sistema Único de Saúde*, São Paulo, Hucitec.

Ciompi, L. (1980), 'The natural history of schizophrenia in the long term', *British Journal of Psychiatry*, 136, 413-420.

Da Matta, R. (1979), *Carnavais, malandros e heróis: para uma sociologia do dilema brasileiro*, Rio de Janeiro, Zahar.

Davidson, L. (2003), *Living outside mental illness: Qualitative research of recovery in schizophrenia*, New York, New York University Press.

Davidson, L. and McGlashan, T.H. (1997), 'The varied outcomes of schizophrenia'. *Canadian Journal of Psychiatry*, 42 (1), 34-43.

Delgado, P.G. *et al.* (2001), 'O Ministério da Saúde e a saúde mental no Brasil: panorama da última década', in Ministério da Saúde, *III Conferência Nacional de Saúde Mental: Caderno de textos*, Brasília, Ministério da Saúde.

Enciclopédia do Mundo Contemporâneo (2000), Rio de Janeiro/São Paulo, Terceiro Milênio/Publifolha.

Fleury, S. (org) (1997), *Saúde e democracia: a luta do CEBES*, São Paulo, Lemos Editorial.

Lin, K.M. and Kleinman, A.M. (1988), 'Psychopathology and clinical course of schizophrenia: A cross-cultural perspective', *Schizophrenia Bulletin*, 14 (4), 555-567.

McGlashan, T.H. (1988), 'A selective review of recent North American long-term follow-up studies of schizophrenia', *Schizophrenia Bulletin*, 14 (4), 515-542.

Ministério da Saúde/Coordenação Geral de Saúde Mental (2003–04), *Saúde mental no SUS*. Informativo da Saúde Mental III (13) Fev 2004. Brasília, Ministério da Saúde.

O Globo (2003) (daily newspaper), Rio de Janeiro.

Oliveira, F. (1976), *Questionando a economia brasileira: a crítica da razão dualista*, Seleções CEBRAP 1, São Paulo, CEBRAP.

Pinheiro, R e Mattos, RA (2001), *O sentidos da integralidade na atenção e no cuidado à saúde*, Rio de Janeiro, IMS/UERJ/ABRASCO.

Ramon, S. (1987), 'The making of a professional culture: Professionals in psychiatry in Britain and Italy since 1945', in L. Hangais and S. Mangen, *Doing cross-national research* 3, Aston University, Birmingham.

Scull, A.T. (1984), *Decarceration: Community treatment and the deviant – a radical view*, Cambridge, Polity Press.

Souza, M.F. (2001a), *A Cor-Agem do PSF*, São Paulo, Hucitec.

Souza, M.F. (2001b), *Agentes comunitários de saúde: choque de povo*, São Paulo, Hucitec.

Souza, M.F. (org) (2002), *Os sinais vermelhos do PSF*, São Paulo, Hucitec.

UNICEF (1978), *Cuidados primários em saúde. Relatório da Conferência Internacional sobre Cuidados Primários em Saúde*, Alma-Ata, URSS. Brasília, 1979.

UNICEF (1998), *The state of the world's children*, New York, UNICEF.

Vasconcelos, E.M. (1992), *The new alienists of the poor: Implementing community mental health policies in Brazil: 1978–1989*, PhD thesis, London School of Economics.

Vasconcelos, E.M. e Furtado, T (eds) (1997), *Saúde Mental e Desinstitucionalização: Reinventado Serviços*, Cadernos n.o 7 do Instituto de Psiquiatria da UFRJ, Rio de Janeiro, IPUB.

Vasconcelos, E.M. (ed.) (1999), *Transversões – Saúde Mental, Desinstitucionalização e Abordagens Psicossociais*, Série 'Periódicos de Pesquisa do Programa de Pós-Graduação da Escola de Serviço Social da UFRJ', N.o I ano I, Rio de Janeiro, UFRJ.

Vasconcelos, E.M. (ed.) (2000), *Saúde mental e serviço social: o desafio da subjetividade e interdisciplinaridade*, São Paulo, Cortez.

Vasconcelos, E.M. (2002), *Complexidade e Pesquisa Interdisciplinar: epistemologia e metodologia operativa*, Petrópolis, Vozes.

Vasconcelos, E.M. (2003), *O poder que brota da dor e da opressão: empowerment, sua história, teorias e estratégias*, São Paulo, Paulus.

Velho, G. (1981), *Individualismo e cultura*, Rio de Janeiro, Zahar.

Warner, R. (1985), *Recovery from schizophrenia: Psychiatry and political economy*, London, Routledge and Kegan Paul.

Weingarten, R. (2001), *O movimento de usuários em saúde mental nos Estados Unidos: história, processos de ajuda e suporte mútuos e militância*, editado por E.M. Vasconcelos *et al.*, Rio de Janeiro, Projeto Transversões e Instituto Franco Basaglia.

Chapter 8

Developing Self-defined Social Approaches to Madness and Distress

Peter Beresford

This discussion starts from a basic premise. What might understandings of 'mental health' issues, policy and practice look like, if they were based on an inclusive model of knowledge? What might the effects be of including in debates viewpoints which have not always adequately been addressed before? The particular (traditionally marginalised) perspective and source of knowledge on which this discussion focuses is that of mental health service users/survivors. Mental health service users have long been a significant knowledge source, in the sense that they have been drawn into research processes like surveys and trials. But their primary role has been as a *data source*. Their views, experience and perceptions have been interpreted and fed into structures of understanding established by clinicians, policymakers, researchers and academics. Here the concern is with service users as active participants and co-constructers of models and thinking about 'mental health' issues and the implications this may have for our broader understanding of these.

Including Mental Health Service Users'/Survivors' Perspectives

It should be made clear, however, that the aim here is not to reject or ignore what may have gone before, but to try and consider what the impact might be of including on equal terms, perspectives and knowledge sources which up until now may have been allowed a very restricted role in the construction of 'mental health' ideas and praxis. It is also worthwhile to remember that mental health service users/survivors may not be the only perspective that has tended to be overlooked. Some commentators might, for example, argue that those of 'carers' have not been afforded adequate, serious or critical consideration. A case might also be made that the perspectives of face-to-face mental health practitioners (other than psychiatrists) have also tended to be granted a very restricted role in debates and theoretical developments.

Of course, developing a new framework for understanding, based on synthesising old and new perspectives will demand a complex process of review and reconsideration, testing and modifying existing understandings in the light of the implications of other viewpoints. We need to keep this process in mind, but it is not one we can take forward adequately here. Rather, here the aim is to set out some possibilities emerging from the experience, knowledge and ideas of service users and to consider their implications for theory and action in the field of 'mental health' and in relation to social understandings of 'mental health' issues.

There are two particular reasons for focusing on service users/survivors here. First, while they have traditionally been excluded and devalued, both generally in society and specifically in the formation of mental health thinking, this situation has begun fundamentally to change. More recently, the viewpoints and experience of service users, as part of a more general shift to public policy based on consumerist and active citizenship models, have been afforded much greater significance. Government commitments to increased 'user involvement'; 'partnership' and 'empowerment' have developed in many areas of policy, practice, services, research and evaluation. This pattern has extended to the field of mental health. The emergence of service users'/survivors' own movement and self-organisation, at national and international levels, has both been supported by this development and given it considerable added force. Thus there is now a definite rhetorical commitment to the involvement of service users and their perspectives and growing pressure for this to be acted on in practice.

The second reason why it is likely to be helpful to focus on the perspectives of mental health service users/survivors, is the current renewal of interest in social approaches to 'mental health issues' more generally. This book is itself a sign of this, as is the recent establishment of the Social Perspectives Network (SPN/TOPSS, 2002). Mental health service users and their organisations have generally tended to embrace more socially based approaches, although this has not always been explicit and service users have frequently at the same time, retained medicalised terminology and frameworks.

Medical models, however, have predominated in the field of psychiatry/mental health, as the language itself makes clear. The core and founding concept of modern psychiatric provision and professions is that of 'mental illness' and of service users/patients being 'mentally ill'. Whether this is presented in terms of 'mental health', 'mental health problems' or 'mental health issues', the core concept underlying policy and provision has continued to be that of 'mental illness'. This continues to be a powerful concept, which still holds considerable political, professional, public and personal authority. On the basis of an ever-expanding range and number of diagnostic categories following from this concept, service users may be subjected to compulsory 'treatment'; physical constraint and other restrictions on their rights.

Such an approach represents a medicalised individual model for the understanding and explanation of mental health service users/survivors, as well as, of their experience, circumstances, feelings and perceptions. This is essentially a *deficit* model, which is based on assumptions of the inherent deficiency and pathology of 'the mentally ill'. It conceptualises people's thoughts, emotions and behaviour as defective and inadequate and has strongly encouraged a quest for bio-chemical and genetic explanations and responses to them – so far with little evidence of long term effectiveness or success.

Addressing the Social

While the medical model of 'mental illness' continues to predominate in mental health policy, provision and analysis, it is not the only model in operation. In the current edition of a definitive text on this subject, five conceptual models in psychiatry are identified in all. These are: the disease, psychodynamic, behavioural, cognitive and social models (Tyrer and Steinberg, 2003). Defining social models, the authors argue that:

> All social models in psychiatry have the same fundamental premise. They regard the wider influence of social forces as more important than other influences as causes or precipitants of mental illness (Tyrer and Steinberg, 2003: 87).

The authors identify three central tenets of 'the social model'. These are that:

- Mental disorder is often triggered by life events that appear to be independent
- Social forces linked to class, occupational status and social role are the precipitants of mental disorder
- People with mental disorder often become and remain disordered because of societal influences (Tyrer and Steinberg, 2003: 87).

This analysis seems to hold and still seems to be reflected in recent and current professional discussions of social models of 'mental health', such as Duggan *et al.* with others (2002). This, however, raises two important points in the context of the present discussion. The first concerns the nature of traditional social models of mental health. The second concerns the emergence of a different approach to a social model.

Historically, a social approach or understanding in mental health and other areas of social policy has been taken primarily to mean taking into account social as well as individual factors that may be linked with certain activities, behaviours or conditions. Thus there may be social as well as individual explanations for a wide range of social problems and phenomena, ranging from poverty and drug addiction, to homelessness and unemployment. Such social approaches tend to place an emphasis on 'nurture' rather than 'nature', highlighting the ways in which the individual may be affected by the social world in which they live and by social forces operating within it. More recently, there has also been a developing discussion about the interrelations between the two; the individual and the social, which has been embodied particularly in interest in 'agency' (what the individual actor can and does do in any setting to influence what happens to them) and 'structure' (the social system in which they live and the influences and constraints it imposes on them).

One feature of such traditional social approaches has particular significance for an idea like 'mental illness'. While they may emphasise explanatory factors outside the individual as well as within him or her, they do not necessarily challenge underpinning conceptual frameworks which may be involved. They may simply relocate the explanation for them. Thus the cause(s) of the individual's 'mental illness' or 'disorder' may now be seen to lie (at least in part) in the wider world, but as 'mentally ill', the individual is still deemed to be problematic and defective. The individual model of 'mental illness' remains unchallenged. This is certainly the model that Tyrer and Steinberg (2003) outline.

Reconceiving the Social

However, some mental health service users/survivors and their organisations, do not take the idea of 'mental illness' for granted, but instead have rejected or sought to challenge it (Curtis *et al.*, 2003). So far explicit discussion of social approaches to mental health issues among mental health service users/survivors is at a relatively early stage. Recently, however, increased interest among survivors in the disabled people's movement, recognition of common concerns and the development of some joint activities with disabled people, have led to an increasing awareness of and interest in the well developed philosophy of the disabled people's movement.

This philosophy has been based on the social model of disability. This social model challenges the idea of the disabled individual's definition as inherently inadequate or defective. It has been developed by disabled people themselves as part of the international disabled people's movement. The social model of disability is a complex and developing idea. It is constantly being critiqued and re-evaluated by disabled people and disabled commentators (Corker and Shakespeare, 2002; Barnes, *et al.*, 2002; Barnes and Mercer, 2004). Its key feature is that it draws a distinction between 'impairment' and 'disability'. Impairment is taken to be the actual or perceived absence or functional limitation of a limb or sense. Disability is defined as the negative societal response to people with (perceived) impairments (Oliver, 1996). Disability therefore is conceived of as a form of social oppression, linked with, but certainly not necessarily following from impairment. The social model of disability has also highlighted two other key concepts: *barriers* and *rights*.

Disabled people have highlighted the ways in which the creation and maintenance of social and other barriers has denied them equality. The disabled peoples' movement has emphasised the centrality of discrimination at both institutional and individual levels. It has highlighted how such barriers have operated to segregate, exclude, subordinate and marginalise disabled people in all areas of their lives, including education, employment, income, leisure and social and political life. It has identified environmental, cultural and attitudinal barriers.

Instead of framing their difficulties in terms of individual health and welfare 'needs', disabled activists and theoreticians have seen the way forward to challenge disability in terms of securing disabled people's civil and human rights (Campbell and Oliver, 1996). This has led to fundamental changes in understandings of and responses to disability. It has led in the UK to the passing and extension of anti-discrimination legislation, the Disability Discrimination Act (1995); the setting up of the Disability Rights Commission and the introduction as mandatory of 'direct payment' schemes (Community Care [Direct Payments] Act, 1996), putting disabled people in control of their own support requirements.

Instead of framing their demands in terms of personal 'care' disabled people have argued their right to access support to enable them to live 'independently'. Direct payments make it possible for disabled people to work out what they want in order to live their lives as closely as they can, to the way they want; recruiting and managing their own support workers. Direct payments have developed as part of the international 'independent living' movement. Disabled people define independent living as meaning having the support to live their life as far as possible on equal terms to non-disabled people, rather than meaning to 'stand on your own two feet' (without support) or necessarily to live on your own in your own home. The emphasis instead is on choice and control.

These developments in the context of 'disability' have increasing ramifications for mental health service users/survivors and those working with them. First, many mental health service users are included in the administrative/welfare category of disabled people and are therefore eligible not only for disability benefits, but also the safeguards and opportunities provided by the recently established legislative and policy provisions following from the social model of disability. This comes at the same time as, by contrast, the rights of mental health service users are being seen as being at increasing risk, with political and media emphasis on the 'dangerousness' of mental health service users, 'protecting the public' and proposals to extend compulsory 'treatment' 'into the community'.

Reconnected the Personal with the Social

Survivor discussions about their lives and experience tend to accent the *holistic* nature of their situation. This includes and interconnects the physical, mental (emotional and perceptual), spiritual, social and political. In this sense they go much further than traditional 'psychosocial' approaches to 'mental health' issues, which have sought to focus attention on both the personal/psychological and the social/structural. Here the emphasis of survivors is on the complex (non-medicalised) interrelations of ourselves, our lives, our minds, our bodies and our environments.

It is important to remember that the increasing interest in social approaches to understanding madness and distress does not neglect or underplay personal and psychological issues. This has been a criticism made of the development of the social model of disability, where it has been argued that the focus on the social response to impairment has sometimes been at the expense of consideration of the impairment itself; and where insufficient attention is felt to have been paid to the interrelations between individual impairment and societal reaction. A strong and developing discussion has developed which has focused on these issues and which has sought to highlight the personal and experiential nature and consequences of both impairment and disability (Crow, 1996; Thomas, 2002a and 2002b).

This is an important reminder that social understandings, like that developing about madness and distress, have such a capacity and that a concern with the social need not overlook (or be at the expense of) the personal and individual. Thus survivors in their own discussions, both published and unpublished, have developed a rights and socially based discourse about issues like social exclusion, unemployment and compulsory 'treatment', at the same time as developing their own and other people's understandings of ideas of 'self-management', self-help, spirituality and complementary therapies, in the context of mental health policy, practice, learning and research. In this author's view, one of the qualities that has always characterised the discussions and campaigning of mental health service users/survivors in the UK, is their interest in both the personal and the social; in personal and political empowerment.

Developing the Social Model

So far, the social model of disability is not fully consistent with the experience and situation of mental health service users/survivors and has not yet been adequately related to them. However, it is possible to see that their rights and needs may be readily framed in similar terms, especially if 'impairment' is also understood as a social construction. Mental health service users/survivors face a wide range of barriers, exclusions and discriminations. They are also a group whose rights may not only be restricted arbitrarily because of their relative powerlessness. There are also routine provisions to restrict their rights as part of the traditional policy approach to dealing with them (Rogers and Pilgrim, 2001). While historically the focus has tended to be on mental health service users/survivors' personal difficulties, these social circumstances and restrictions are now well evidenced (Sayce, 2000).

While, as has been said, discussion among mental health service users/survivors about a social model approach has been limited, it has implicitly informed much of their thinking and activities. As early as 1987, at its founding conference Survivors Speak Out, the pioneering organisation controlled by psychiatric system survivors produced a 'Charter of Needs and Demands' which were agreed unanimously. These prioritised the value of people's first hand experience, the rights of service users, the provision of non-medicalised services and the ending of discrimination against people with experience of using mental health services (Survivors Speak Out, 1987).

Some of the most groundbreaking developments that survivors have pioneered most clearly connect to such a new social understanding of mental health issues. This is exemplified by the development of the international hearing voices movement and in the UK of the Hearing Voices Network. Instead of accepting the diagnosis 'schizophrenia', the emphasis has been on trying to make sense of hearing voices both at an individual personal and societal level, learning to understand and deal with it better (Romme and Escher, 1993; Coleman and Smith, 1997; Coleman, 1999). The same has been true of developments relating to self-harm and eating distress. Self-harm has been reconceived as a coping strategy and a frequently appropriate response to difficult, hostile and inappropriate experiences, like childhood sexual abuse and domestic violence. (Pembroke, 1994; Arnold, Magill 1996; National Self-Harm Network, 1998; Pacitti, 1998; Trump, 2001). Survivors have reconceived 'anorexia nervosa' as 'eating distress', demedicalising the phenomenon and highlighting its social, cultural and gender relations (Pembroke, 1992). In all these areas of formal 'diagnosis', survivors have made it possible for people to re-examine themselves and their difficulties in broader social, cultural and political context, in the light of shared experience, without stigma or negative stereotyping. They have also provided a practical basis for the development of collective action, mutual aid, support and self-help.

Mental health service users'/survivors' own innovative ideas and developments over recent years, offer a basis for a new social approach to 'mental health', or as many survivors prefer to call it, 'madness and distress', that is consistent with an anti-discriminatory, anti-oppressive and rights based philosophy. A range of elements for such an approach can now be identified from existing experience, particularly that developed by service users/survivors and their organisations. These elements have emerged in the discussions taking place in local service user groups, among service users and their organisations, among activists, on survivor websites, in newsletters and other so-called survivor 'grey literature' and to a lesser extent in the conventional mental health literature. Most if not all of these elements already have a track record of development. What generally has not yet happened, is for them to be put together as part of an adequately resourced and supported strategic approach to 'mental health' policy and practice development and reform. Such elements can be seen to include first, a series of underpinning principles or values; second, a range of constituents which shape the proposed support and provision and third, a number of broader commitments which are likely to be required for such an approach to be achievable (Beresford, 2003). This discussion will outline all these elements, but focus particularly on the second; the constituents of socially based support and services.

The principles or values of such a socially based system are likely to include:

- Being rights based and anti-discriminatory, rather than focusing narrowly on the individual
- Valuing self-management and self-support (Hooks, 1993; Faulkner and Layzell, 2000)
- A commitment to anti-oppressive practice
- Supporting race equality and cultural diversity
- Prioritising advocacy and self-advocacy
- Minimising compulsion in the psychiatric services by prioritising prevention, rapid and appropriate support and advanced directives
- Breaking the bad/mad link that continues to be a driver in mental health policy and provision
- Prioritising participation in the development, management and running of policy and services
- Equalising power relations between service providers and service users in services and support.

Components for Socially Based Services and Support

Much more developmental work needs to be done before there is a clear, agreed and well evidenced picture of what mental health service users/survivors see as the essentials for appropriate and effective services and support. But from discussions and developments that have already taken place, an outline of key components can be sketched out as a basis for further discussion and development. Components that are repeatedly identified include:

- Services and support based on self-defined needs and rights
- Self run services
- Valuing holistic and complementary approaches to support
- Extended schemes for personal support
- User-led training and education
- Encouraging community development approaches in mental health
- Developing new roles and approaches in mental health services and support.

It is helpful to look at each of these in more detail.

Services and Support Based on Self-defined Needs and Rights

Rights and the meeting and safeguarding of people's civil and human rights necessarily play a much more central role in a mental health system based on an anti-discriminatory social model. The mental health system has traditionally been based on ideas of 'need'. This approach has tended to have a number of shortcomings. It has generally followed from the definitions and judgements of professionals and organisations employing a medicalised individual model. This approach has emphasised people's inabilities and deficiencies, rather than their capacity. In order to qualify for support, people have had to demonstrate their deficiencies. This has worked against preventive approaches to madness and distress. It frequently means that people cannot access a small amount of support needed to enable them to maintain their lives and activities and that these are then put in jeopardy.

Moving to a model based on self-definition of needs and rights makes it possible, with appropriate advocacy, information and support, for service users to be able to identify what support they would want to do the things they would like to do. This was the aspiration at the heart of the care management and care programme approach introduced in 1993 with the Community Care reforms.

To work, this is likely to require:

- Independent, reliable and accessible information
- Independent advocacy, including peer advocacy and support for self-advocacy
- Independent (non-medicalised) assessment (Leader, 1995).

Disabled people's organisations have established precedents here, developing roles, training and accreditation enabling service users to provide such support on an independent basis, informed by shared experience.

Self-run Services

Research has indicated that mental health and other service users especially value the services and support provided by user controlled services (Barnes, Mercer and Morgan, 2000 and 2001). Mental health service users have been seeking to develop their own non-medicalised services for at least two decades. Some pioneering initiatives have been established (Lindow, 1994 and 1999). These include safe and crisis houses, employment and environmental schemes, counselling, advocacy, information and advice services and so on. However, service users and their organisations have found it very difficult to get the funding and other support to develop these initiatives on any scale. Their status has often been precarious and valued services have closed through failure to refund them. Service users are thus frequently denied this choice and even where such services are available, mainstream services are sometimes unaware of their existence and don't refer service users to them. Government has argued for the importance of diversity in service provision and highlighted an expanded role for the voluntary sector. As part of this aspiration, the important, valued and specific contribution of user controlled/self-run services needs to be recognised. The insecurity and under-funding of such services means that their skilled and experienced workers often have to move on to conventional services, to ensure some reliability of income and security in their own lives.

A strategic approach to supporting the development of such user controlled and self-run services is needed. This requires the allocation of specific (secure) funding and the independent evaluation of such provision. Such services also offer important employment, training and career opportunities for mental health service users/survivors. More support and evaluation will be needed to maximise these opportunities and to enhance skill development and career opportunities for service users.

Valuing Holistic and Complementary Approaches to Support

The medical base of mental health policy and thinking; the tendency to separate the mind from the body, has encouraged medicalised 'treatment' responses to people included as mental health service users. This has been reinforced by the bureaucratic tendency to organise and compartmentalise according to policy and administrative concerns, rather than on the basis of individual lives, rights, wants and needs.

Traditional 'scientific' prejudices have also discouraged the development and application of the wide range of complementary therapies available. This has begun to change. User controlled and voluntary organisations as well as private practitioners are increasingly offering such approaches. They are also entering mainstream statutory services. They are valued by many service users/survivors. They reflect and are sympathetic to service users' interest in holistic and non-medicalised responses to their experience and feelings (Faulkner, 1997; Faulkner and Layzell, 2000). But they are far from being a routine option for many service users, especially not for the majority on low income. Such services are particularly suited and receptive to an holistic approach to madness and emotional and mental distress. Policy and provision based on a rights based social model is likely to develop a more holistic approach to the rights and needs of service users. This includes:

- Seeing the individual as a person, not a collection of problems, symptoms or deficits
- Integrating policies; recognising the interrelation of different aspects of the person's life and connecting policies to fit these. It is not enough to see policy and provision for mental health service users as the sole concern of the National Health Service. The wide range of relevant policy areas, including income maintenance, public transport, leisure and recreation, education and employment, will also need to be fully taken into account and audited against the inclusive and participatory goals of a socially based approach to madness and distress
- Giving equal recognition to complementary approaches to healing valued by service users, enabling them to be evaluated in appropriate ways.

Extending Self-run Schemes for Personal Support

The main way in which the disabled people's movement in the UK has been able to advance the idea of 'independent living' based on a social model of disability, has been through the introduction of 'direct payments' or 'self-run personal assistance' schemes. What these mean essentially, is that the individual service user, after assessment, receives an allocation of state funding directly themselves, with which they are then able to purchase the 'package of support' which *they* want, to meet their support needs as they define them. Disabled people have commonly used this money to employ 'personal assistants (who they hire and fire) to meet their support requirements. So far, such direct payments schemes, which have subsequently been extended by legislation to become a mandatory option for a wider range of service users, including many mental health service users, have represented the strongest expression of 'user controlled' support for health and social care service users (Kestenbaum, 1995; Hasler *et al.*, 1998).

As yet, a relatively small number of mental health service users are accessing direct payments, but such schemes are rapidly gaining in support and interest from mental health service users. They make it possible for service users to reassess their support needs in non-medicalised terms and secure the kind of assistance which they find helpful. This includes personal assistance; out of hours help; help with day to day tasks (like cooking, going out and shopping), counselling, advice and 'talking therapies' (Spandler and Vick, 2004).

Such self-run personal assistance schemes do not offer a panacea and they should be seen as an option, rather than the only approach available to service users. However, survivors receiving them, report fewer in-patient hospital stays and the possibility of avoiding crises through having support in advance of their situation worsening.

If such schemes are to work for the wide range of mental health service users who are now entitled to them, then experience strongly indicates that local user controlled organisations need to be established and properly funded to offer the back up, financial and technical support and advice to enable *every* service user (regardless of their experience and expertise) to run such a scheme without it being burdensome or difficult. The evidence from direct payments schemes for disabled people also highlights that the health of people receiving such schemes tends to improve and that they gain transferable skills which can, for example, help them return to employment if they want to.

User-led Training and Education

Service users, their organisations; progressive practitioners and service organisations, have long argued that involving service users in staff education and training can play a crucial role in improving service cultures and making them more 'user centred' and social model based (Hastings and Crepaz-Keay, 1995). Even on a piecemeal basis, the introduction of 'user training', the development of a growing number of user trainers and the development of 'training for user trainers' have all made a valuable impact on mental health provision and practice. What is still needed is a coherent and systematic approach to user involvement in mental health training which goes far beyond bringing in service users to offer one-off sessions on their personal experience. The new three year social work qualification, introduced in 2003, requires service user involvement in *all* aspects of professional education and it is such a coherent approach which is needed across mental health occupations, professions and disciplines (Levin, 2004). Such an approach includes user involvement in recruitment, curriculum development, teaching, assessment and accreditation. It draws on materials produced by mental health service users and their organisations to complement other sources of learning material. Such materials are now increasingly being produced.

Encouraging Community Development Approaches

Mental health policy and provision have generally tended to operate in relation to the individual. An anti-oppressive social model approach highlights the need to address collective and structural issues too. Initiatives which seek to enable people to come together to achieve change and support together have a long and successful track record in this field (Rogers and Pilgrim, 2001). Therapeutic communities can be seen to be located at one end of this continuum. This includes for example, the pioneering work of therapeutic communities based on principles of social psychiatry (for example, the Henderson Hospital); of prisons like Grendon Underwood, which have offered therapeutic and group support; as well as group work and group therapy more generally. At the other end of the continuum can be seen to be the collective action and self-organisation of mental health service users/survivors, including pioneering initiatives like Survivors Speak Out and the United Kingdom Advocacy Network (UKAN). Self-organisation, as we have also seen, can also provide the basis for mental health service users to develop and provide their own user-led services and support.

Community development approaches, therefore, are likely to have a particular contribution to offer in social approaches to madness and distress inspired by mental health service users themselves. They make it possible to:

- Reach out and involve a diverse range of service users
- Challenge isolation by operating pro-actively rather than reactively
- Engage with and understand service users in the context of their own communities (of locality, interest and identity)
- Engage and reinforce the abilities and capacities of service users
- Support collective working
- Bring the strengths of mutual aid and support to bear in the context of collective action for change
- Support self and mutual empowerment.

Community development approaches have frequently emphasised the importance of involvement and empowerment. They are especially helpful where service users and service user organisations employ them and have an effective say in how they are used.

Developing New Roles and Approaches in Mental Health Services and Support

Almost all the roles associated with mental health policy and practice have their origins in medicalised individual approaches to treatment and understanding. This is not a comment on their value or legitimacy. Mental health service users still most often comment on whether their psychiatrist, social worker or CPN (community psychiatric nurse) is a 'good' or a 'bad' one, according to the nature of the individual worker, rather than according to the inherent nature of the role. All the occupational and professional roles associated with the mental health system are more or less based on a model of 'mental illness'. This includes social work (despite its commitment to social approaches) and psychology – even if their analysis, modelling and interventions are different from those of mainstream psychiatry.

However, in the context of developing discussions about a social model of madness and distress and with the advent of self-run services, complementary approaches, schemes for personal support and new approaches to self-management and self-support, it is now particularly timely to explore new roles and new approaches to practice and occupational roles. This has already happened in the context of disability where new roles and services have been pioneered by the disabled people's movement. Here services not conceived in medicalised terms or in terms of rehabilitation, have developed over the last few years. This has resulted in new approaches to training as well as distinct new roles, usually based on the recruitment of people with direct experience of disability. This includes roles concerned with providing personal assistance, social and housing advice, peer advocacy and counselling and assessment. In some cases this has led to certificated training programmes as well as the emergence of recognised new roles.

This has also begun to happen in the field of mental health. However, this is a development which would now benefit from being taken forward in association with mental health service users and their organisations in a much more strategic and systematic way. There are already a number of emerging roles to build on and develop, for example:

- service user telephone helpline workers
- non-medicalised crisis and safe-house workers
- peer advocates
- employment and employment support workers
- non-medicalised support workers.

Such roles need to be explored, training developed (and training materials produced) and schemes for accreditation established, to create a range of new roles alongside traditional mental health ones. There is also a place for developing new materials and input to support traditional roles (for example, in social work, occupational therapy and nursing) to address and include a social model of madness and distress and to explore its implications for the development of conventional practice (Beresford, 2004).

There has been discussion and developments have taken place in all these areas internationally over the last 15 to 20 years. But progress in the UK has been slow and patchy. There is unlikely to be any real shift to a socially based mental health system without broader changes in attitudes and priorities. To make this possible, a number of broader commitments are likely to be required. These are likely to include commitments to:

- Strengthening user controlled organisations
- More support for self-education and prevention
- A greater emphasis on societal education and prevention
- Valuing user experience in the workforce
- Continuity of support
- Supporting user research and evaluation
- The improvement of quality based on developing user-defined standards
- More effective anti-discrimination legislation.

Then we may begin to see the potential of a rights based approach to mental health issues, both to prevent problems arising, ensure appropriate support for those who continue to be affected and to challenge the discrimination and barriers that currently continue to marginalise and exclude mental health service users/survivors.

References

Arnold, L. and Magill, A. (1996), *Working With Self Injury: A Practical Guide*, Basement Project.

Barnes, C., Mercer, G. and Morgan, H. (2000), *Creating Independent Futures: An Evaluation of Services led by Disabled People, Stage One Report*, Leeds: The Disability Press.

Barnes, C., Mercer, G. and Morgan, H. (2001), *Creating Independent Futures: An Evaluation of Services led by Disabled People, Stage Three Report*, Leeds: The Disability Press.

Barnes, C., Oliver, M. and Barton, L. (eds) (2002), *Disability Studies Today*, Cambridge: Polity Press.

Barnes, C. and Mercer, G. (eds) (2004), *Implementing The Social Model of Disability: Theory and research*, Leeds: Disability Press.

Beresford, P. (2003), *Alt MH: Developing a new vision for mental health policy and provision*, Position Paper, Mental Health Task Group, Choice, Responsiveness and Equity Consultation, London, Department of Health.

Beresford, P. (2004), 'Reframing the Nurse's Role through a Social Model Approach: A Rights Based Approach to Workers' Development', *The Journal of Psychiatric and Mental Health Nursing*.

Campbell, J. and Oliver, M. (1996), *Disability Politics: Understanding our Past, Changing our Future*, London: Routledge.

Coleman, R. and Smith, M. (1997), *Working With Voices!! Victim to Victor*, Runcorn: Handsell Publications.

Coleman, R. (1999), 'Hearing voices and the politics of oppression', in Newnes, C., Holmes, G. and Dunn, C. (eds), *This Is Madness: A Critical Look at Psychiatry and the Future of Mental Health Services*, Ross-on-Wye: PCCS Books.

Corker, M. and Shakespeare, T. (eds) (2002), *Disability/Postmodernity*, London: Continuum.

Crow, L. (1996), 'Including all our lives: Renewing the social model of disability', in C. Barnes and E. Mercer (eds), *Exploring The Divide, Illness and disability*, Leeds: The Disability Press, pp. 55-73.

Curtis, T., Dellar, R., Leslie, E. and Watson, B. (eds) (2003), *The Madpride Anthology* (previously published as, *Mad Pride: A Celebration of Mad Culture*), London: Chipamunka Publishing.

Duggan, M. with Cooper, A. and Foster, J., 'Modernising the social model in mental health', a discussion paper presented to the Social Perspectives Network/Topss (England) meeting, Leeds 2002.

Faulkner, A. (1997), *Knowing Our Own Minds: A Survey of How People in Emotional Distress Take Control of their Lives*, London: The Mental Health Foundation.

Faulkner, A. and Layzell, S. (2000), *Strategies For Living: A Report of User-led Research into People's Strategies for Living with Mental Distress*, London: The Mental Health Foundation.

Hasler, F., Campbell, J. and Zarb, J. (1998), *Direct Routes to Independence*, London: Policy Studies Institute.

Hastings, M. and Crepaz-Keay, D. (1995), *The Survivors' Guide To Training Approved Social Workers*, London: Central Council for Education and Training in Social Work (CCETSW).

Hooks, B. (1993), *Sisters Of The Yam: Black Women and Self-recovery*, London: Turnaround.

Kestenbaum, A. (1995), *Independent Living: A Review of Findings and Experience*, York: Joseph Rowntree Foundation.

Leader, A. (1995), *Direct Power: A Resource Pack for People Who Want to Develop their Own Care Plans and Support Networks*, Brighton: Pavilion Publishing.

Levin, E. (2004), 'Involving Service Users and Carers in Social Work Education', Resource Guide No 2, March, London: Social Care Institute for Excellence (SCIE).

Lindow, V. (1994), *Self-Help Alternatives to Mental Health Services*, London: Mind Publications.

Lindow, V. (1999), 'Survivor controlled alternatives to psychiatric services', in Newnes, C., Holmes, G. and Dunn, C. (eds), *This Is Madness: A Critical Look at Psychiatry and the Future of Mental Health Services*, Ross on Wye: PCCS Books.

National Self-Harm Network (1998), *The Hurt Yourself Less Workbook*, London: National Self-Harm Network.

Oliver, M. (1996), *Understanding Disability: From Theory to Practice*, Basingstoke: Macmillan.

Pacitti, R. (1998), 'Damage Limitation', *Nursing Times* (Self Harm) **94**(27), 8 July, 36-39.

Pembroke, L. (1992), *Eating Distress, Perspectives from Personal Experience*, Chesham: Survivors Speak Out.

Pembroke, L. (ed.) (1994), *Self-Harm: Perspectives from Personal Experience*, London: Survivors Speak Out.

Rogers, A. and Pilgrim, D. (2001), *Mental Health Policy in Britain*, Second edn, Basingstoke: Palgrave Macmillan.

Romme, M.A.J. and Escher, A.D.M.A.C. (eds) (1993), *Accepting Voices*, London: Mind.

Sayce, L. (2000), *From Psychiatric Patient to Citizen: Overcoming Discrimination and Social Exclusion*, Basingstoke: Macmillan.

Spandler, H. and Vick, N. (2004), *Implementing Direct Payments in Mental Health: An Evaluation*, London: Health and Social Care Advisory Service (HASCAS).

Social Perspectives Network/Training Organisation for the Personal Social Services England (2002), 'New Network To Promote "Social Model" of Mental Health', in the *News Release*, Leeds, 14 February 2002.

Survivors Speak Out (1987), *Charter of Needs And Demands – Edale Conference Charter*, London: Survivors Speak Out.

Thomas, C. (2002a), 'A journey around the social model', in M. Corker and T. Shakespeare (eds), *Disability/Postmodernity: Embodying Disability Theory*, London: Continuum.

Thomas, C. (2002b), 'Disability theory: Key ideas, issues and thinkers', in C. Barnes, M. Oliver and Barton, L. (eds), *Disability Studies Today*, Cambridge: Polity Press.

Trump, A. (2001), 'Making Meaning from Tragedy: Sharon Lefevre', *Psychminded* (www.psychminded.co.uk).

Tyrer, P. and Steinberg, D. (2003), *Models For Mental Disorder, Conceptual Models in Psychiatry*, Third edn, Chichester: John Wiley & Sons.

Part Four
The Psychosocial:
Experience and Practice

Chapter 9

The Place of Recovery

Jan Wallcraft

The psychosocial challenge to biomedical dominance in mental health, which been ongoing for centuries, is in the 21st century bolstered by broad alliances between psychosocial professionals and academics, the voluntary sector and the service user movement. The recovery paradigm is a unifying factor for this alliance. I will examine here whether recovery is a paradigm in itself or an aspect of other worldviews. People with different perspectives, including those who accept the biomedical model of mental illness, have claimed recovery as part of their model. Is there a 'pure' version of recovery that cannot be co-opted to fit pre-existing views?

I discuss 'recovery' as a concept whose philosophical boundaries and practical implications are still contested, make links between the concept of recovery in mental health and concepts of systemic change and transformation in other areas of scientific enquiry, and draw conclusions as to its potential impact on system change. The concept of recovery, I argue, has transformative implications for the whole of society.

The Recovery Concept

Recovery is not easy to define. Put most simply, it means to get better after a breakdown or a period of mental ill-health or emotional distress. What makes defining recovery complicated is that the language used is inevitably imbued with resonances from differing worldviews. Writers from the biomedical model or from the psychosocial model will define recovery differently, while mental health system survivors will define it differently again, from the perspective of personal empowerment.

Repper and Perkins (2003) have defined recovery from a psychosocial and an empowerment perspective. They describe it as a process rather than a goal. They point to its origins in the writings of people with mental health problems. They argue that recovery is not the same as cure, but is about growing and overcoming challenges; it is a unique, personal and continuing journey rather than an end-point or outcome. Recovery is about taking back control of one's life, whatever the perceived causes of the original problems, and even if distress or disabilities still remain. Thornton (2004) in contrast incorporates recovery into the biomedical model and the acceptance of brain disease such as schizophrenia rather than anything that one has done such as taking drugs or the result of a dysfunctional family.

The different perceptions of the meaning of recovery lead to differing perceptions of how to achieve it. At a national policy level in the UK the recovery concept has been adopted by the National Institute for Mental Health in England (NIMHE) as the goal for which mental health services should be aiming. Some mental health Trusts are now working out the implications of a recovery focus on their work. There is much to learn from the US, where the recovery concept originated and has been debated for longer. In 2003, the President's Freedom Commission on Mental Health recommended a complete reorganisation of the mental health system to make recovery oriented services available to service users and their families and carers (McLean, 2003). He credits this official acceptance of 'recovery' as due to lobbying by the US consumer/survivor movement:

> The consumer/survivor movement has gained momentum in recent years, broadening its coalitions and finding vigorous support for its holistic vision of recovery, as evidenced both in the Surgeon General's 1999 report and the newly released report of the Freedom Commission on Mental Health (McLean, 2003: 48).

McLean argues that 'recovery' resulted from the coming together of the anti-psychiatry ex-patient movement, which began in the 1960s, and the more mainstream 'consumer' movement, beginning in the 1980s. The anti-psychiatry movement was led by those who 'objected to institutionalization and treatments that deprived them of hope, independence and control over their lives' (McLean, 2003). This group are more likely to point to iatrogenic injury caused by medication and to reject diagnostic labelling, while those who call themselves 'consumers' often accept the biomedical model but call for more community support to help them recover. Both groups have called into question medical opinions about the 'biological irreversible chronic nature of their disorder', and along with that, the need to stay on medication for life.

Even the US families' movement, NAMI, who have been generally opposed to any psychosocial challenges to the biomedical model of severe mental illness, are now interested in recovery, judging by the large amount of information and links to recovery sites on some NAMI websites in the US (NAMI Santa Cruz County, 2004). The tentative consensus growing among consumers/survivors and the US families movement about recovery highlights the problem of the weighting of research, policy and funding towards the biomedical discourse, where physical treatments are the central plank, to the detriment of the social and psychological needs of patients.

However, an anti-recovery backlash has come from writers such as Torrey (2001), a prominent US psychiatrist has written and campaigned vigorously for out-patient commitment laws, citing controversial figures about the dangers to society from unmedicated patients in the community. Similar arguments have been common in the UK.

The Debates About 'Recovery' in Britain

Recovery is different from the traditional concept of rehabilitation, which was managed by professionals, usually in a medical setting, and offered limited scope for service users to define their own goals. Diagnostic labels were too likely to influence practitioners in their views of what patients could achieve.

Recovery is now seen as likely to work best in a real world setting, with service users leading the way and service providers helping them to dream their future, plan the steps towards it, and to identify the help they need, such as skills training, along the way. Collaboration, rather than control, is the keyword. For instance, those in the Supported Housing and Recovery Project in Hertfordshire have worked with members of a local user group to design their own self-assessment tools to enable service users to devise their personal development plans (SHARP, 2001).

Despite the increasing acceptance of recovery in national policy, the concept has met with some resistance in Britain, from service users, researchers and clinicians. Some people are wary because they see 'recovery' as transplanted from the US, rather than originating in our own service user/survivor movement. Policy makers who hope to see 'recovery' flourish would be wise to discuss the concept with service user groups until it is fully understood and owned, or a compromise concept emerges. In my view the controversy and debate that the concept of recovery arouses is usually valuable.

Resistance to the concept comes from radical and reformist service users, but especially from those who have been using services over many years. They have good reason to fear that 'recovery' may just be another buzz-word for mental health policy makers that will make little positive impact on their lives.

Many see the concept of recovery as too idealistic and as denying the of power imbalances between service users and professionals. They argue that recovery is meaningless given the social prejudice and discrimination against people with a mental illness label. Service users who see themselves as suffering from an illness or a long-term incurable condition often fear the idea of recovery. The relentless bureaucratic pressures that many long-term service users experience in getting the services and benefits they are entitled to leads them to regard a 'recovery' orientation as essentially a cost-cutting exercise, and they fear being deprived of needed treatment, support and benefits. They fear being prematurely forced into low paid, menial, unpleasant and stressful work, without any reduction of the social stigma of having been labelled 'mentally ill' in the first place. This is likely to be a lose-lose situation for them. Rethink, when it was the National Schizophrenia Fellowship, warned about recovery. They did not want it to become something imposed and raising unrealistic expectations on people who were struggling already with illness, disability and stigma. They saw it as successful if it was inclusive of everyone using mental health services, including their interest group who were likely to be making only small steps towards a fuller life (NSF, 2001).

Survivors or service users, who reject the label of mental illness and see their problems as the direct result of bad experiences, or who locate the problem with social oppression on the basis of their difference, often view the recovery concept as a way of putting the problem back onto the individual (Beresford and Hopton, 2003). They want to see a movement for rights working at a social, economic and political level. Recovery, from this perspective, could be a new way for professionals to treat 'the sick', whilst lining their own pockets and enhancing their own reputations, and could undermine the social model of disability in mental health.

I will argue below that neither of these objections, the 'cost-cutting' objection, or the 'individualising' objection, should prevent 'recovery' being seen as a concept that is essentially service user/survivor friendly. However, for it to be so, it must be owned, defined and used by service users/survivors primarily, as individuals and as self-advocacy groups, and that ownership must be respected by service providers, planners, academics and politicians.

Despite the reservations of many British survivors and service users, others have taken up the notion of recovery with enthusiasm. No Panic, a user led organisation for people who experience anxiety disorders has set up nineteen telephone recovery groups which use telephone conferencing and provide structured support based on cognitive behaviour therapy. This has enabled people who would otherwise be isolated and unable to access services to find the help they need. No Panic followed up the success of the recovery groups by providing volunteer-run befriending groups to help people continue on the road to recovery. Others have benefited directly from the work of US survivors. The Manic Depression fellowship adapted Copeland's (1997) Wellness Action Recovery Plans (WRAP) to create self management planning tools for their members (MDF, 2002), though changing the language to the more UK-friendly 'self-management' (perhaps an indication of resistance to recovery language).

Mental health researchers in the UK often resist the recovery concept as an evangelistic doctrine preached to the sceptical British by enthusiasts from abroad, which is resistant to statistical measurement. Hope, a notion central to recovery, is individual and personal and cannot be given in controlled doses by a doctor or therapist to a patient or client. Yet while 'recovery' is criticised in this way, 'schizophrenia' and 'mental illness', which have also been argued to be concepts based on beliefs rather than grounded in material reality (Boyle, 1996), are usually accepted uncritically in scientific research.

However, a number of Trusts are implementing recovery-oriented services. For example, West Hampshire NHS Trust have trained some staff in Copeland's (1997) WRAP system, and are running groups based on this work. These groups, currently facilitated by nursing staff and clinical psychologists, enable service users to maximise their potential whilst acknowledging the possibility of future crises by writing their own crisis plan. Service users are helped to build their own support networks and develop coping strategies. The vision is that service users will learn skills to co-facilitate WRAP groups and eventually be able to own and run the programme themselves.

Sections of the UK mental health voluntary sector have shown positive interest in the recovery concept. Both Mind and Rethink have carried out investigations of what 'recovery' means to service users and how it can be implemented in service provision (Baker and Strong, 2001; Rethink, 2004). Rethink have called it variously a recovery, an organising and generative idea, an underlying vision, a movement, a journey, and a prize (Rethink, 2004). Under their former name of National Schizophrenia Fellowship they stated that the belief in a positive future is vitally important for everyone involved. In this model there was hope in realistic measure and that it was user led whilst being able to motivate staff (NSF, 2001). Rethink's description of 'recovery; as a uniting and motivating vision' is arguably representative of the more positive responses to the concept in the UK.

Is 'Recovery' a New Paradigm for Mental Health?

It is somewhat surprising that recovery in mental health has been so controversial or that there should be a perceived need for a new paradigm that includes recovery. In most other areas of health, it is not news that the patient may get better, or that recovery should be a desired and expected outcome of treatment. Yet, particularly for people with diagnoses of severe mental illness, such as schizophrenia and manic depression, this has not been the case. Secker (2004) describes the subtle influence on her thinking as a mental health nurse:

> I don't think it was ever made very explicit, but throughout my practice career you felt a certain unspoken hopelessness when someone was given a diagnosis of schizophrenia and you saw your role, to put it a bit bluntly, as helping them to make the best of a bad job … it's just the way we thought in a very taken-for-granted, implicit kind of way – it was another of those certainties, sad but true (Secker, 2004: 34).

The biomedical model goes further than subtle influence on the minds of mental health workers. Schizophrenia has been defined in terms of the inability of patients to recover (Kruger, 2000). In other words, if a patient recovers they probably never actually had the illness in the first place. This circularity of argument indicates that that the diagnosis of schizophrenia is based on a belief system rather than being a clearly defined and refutable scientific hypothesis, to use the Popperian definition of true science (Popper, 1987).

Studies from the 1960s onwards (Ciompi, 1980; Huber *et al.*, 1980; Ogawa *et al.*, 1987; Desisto *et al.*, 1995) show that 50 to 68 per cent of people with schizophrenia do recover, however strict the definition of recovery. Kruger (2000) argues that the evidence base now shows there should be a new paradigm of schizophrenia as a 'prolonged illness with an ameliorating course'.

As Pat Deegan, one of the originators of the recovery concept puts it:

> Recovery is not the privilege of a few exceptional clients. We can now tell people the good news that empirical data indicate most people do recover. Since there is no way to predict who will or will not recover, we should approach each person as being able to recover if given sufficient opportunity to build skills and supports. In this way professionals can stop the iatrogenic wounding of hopelessness and begin working with clients on the transformative journey of recovery (Deegan, 2001: 21).

If over half of people diagnosed with schizophrenia recover despite the psychiatric system treating them as unlikely to do so, then perhaps a recovery orientation, taking into account the individual's pathway through services over time, could achieve far better results. Service users' high levels of expressed dissatisfaction with acute services and the concentration of treatment on medication rather than social support (Johnson *et al.*, 1997; SCMH, 1998; MHF, 2000; Levinson *et al.*, 2003), show that recovery at present, when it does occur, is likely to be a creative achievement by service users who are finding their own ways to survive, find help, and improve their lives (Faulkner and Layzell, 2000) despite low spending on rehabilitation and community services.

In the next section I will make an argument for recovery to be seen as part of a new, more empowering, spiritual and psychosocial conceptualisation of the underpinning knowledge base in mental health.

The Basis for the 'Recovery' Concept in Post-Cartesian, Holistic Science

The concept of recovery has parallels in branches of science other than orthodox medicine. It fits well with the new post-Cartesian, holistic scientific philosophy of complexity and chaos, which has resulted from the work of leading physicists (Michaelson and Wallcraft, 1997).

Pert (1997) describes the deal negotiated with the Pope in the 17th century by Descartes, the philosopher and 'founding father of modern medicine' that gave him access to human bodies for dissection providing he agreed to have nothing to do with the soul, mind or the emotions, which were the realm of the church. This set the direction of Western science thereafter, 'creating the unbalanced situation that is mainstream science as we know it today' (1997: 18). Medical and psychological science was forced to adopt reductionist methodologies, according to which life could be understood by breaking it down to its smallest components and drawing conclusions to apply to the whole, rather than looking at whole systems in their environment, which might challenge Church orthodoxy. Science took charge of the realm of the concrete and rational, leaving mysticism and spirituality, with emotions, thoughts and dreams, to the Church.

Psychiatry has remained to this day largely based on the Cartesian philosophy of science, treating the phenomena of mind as if they were rooted entirely in the physical, and the physical as if it could be understood as pure mechanics. Scientific theories of 'mental illness', a concept with no clear and obvious physical existence or causation, were created in imitation of other branches of medical science.

Boyle (1996) argues that diagnostic labels are more accurately thought of as concepts, not concrete things, yet the way in which they are used confers on them a 'permanence and solidity which is quite unwarranted' (1996: 7). The assumption of the solid and definable reality of schizophrenia is a central plank in the biomedical discourse of psychopathology.

Once schizophrenia had been defined as an incurable biological disease, the idea of recovery was regarded as unrealistic. In this way, 19th and 20th century psychiatrists were protected from criticism if their treatments did not work.

Recovery, I argue, is part of a new scientific discourse which, in its more holistic and post-Cartesian approach, would seem to be more suitable to the understanding of the inner world of human beings, and their responses to their environment. The elements of what helps recovery cannot be isolated and distilled and injected into people in a sterile environment. It is irreducibly complex and must be studied in its complexity. For example, an American study of recovery (Onken *et al.*, 2002) took the domains of recovery for its starting point to be resources/basic needs, choices/self determination, independence, interdependence/connectiveness, and hope. They argue that 'recovery is facilitated or impeded through the dynamic interplay of many forces that are complex, synergistic and linked' (2002: vii).

Complexity theory and holistic systems thinking have been applied to mental health and psychology by a number of writers, including Capra (1983) who argues that the psyche can create 'mental illness' but also heal itself, and argues that recovering from mental distress is a process of inner growth and self-realisation, which is linked to one's emotional, social and cultural environment. Grof and Grof (1989) argue that unusual experiences and states of mind that are diagnosed and treated as mental illness could in many cases be crises of personal spiritual transformation. They argue that traditional psychiatry makes no distinction between psychosis and mysticism and tends to treat all 'nonordinary states of consciousness by suppressive medication' (Grof and Grof, 1989: xi). Spiritual crises, they suggest, may be part of the evolutionary change and growth process for individuals and for humanity as a whole.

Pert (1997) is a neuroscientist whose work on the biochemical basis for the emotions and the immune system crosses Cartesian boundaries and provides a basis for a holistic science of mind and body. She shows that that the body, not just the brain, holds onto traumatic memories. Depression and other forms of mental illness, Pert argues, are linked to traumas that stress the body and disrupt the production of body chemicals, the neurotransmitters, or neuropeptides as she terms them, which regulate the emotions. A person who has suffered repeated stresses without sufficient support to deal with them can get into a chronic state of stress that brings a sensation of constant negative expectation, which can further lead to repetitive and limited patterns of behaviour and responses. She argues that drugs do not solve the problems. They disrupt the natural balance of the feedback loops, which involve many systems and organs, and can cause other physical problems. Holistic therapies such as touch and talking treatments to reduce stress and negative expectations could reverse the process. She provides the science to back the idea that hugs, not drugs, may be the answer to recovery:

> ... each of us has his or her own natural pharmacopoeia – the very finest drugstore available at the cheapest cost – to produce all the drugs we ever need to run our bodymind in precisely the way it was designed to run over centuries of evolution ... Research needs to focus on understanding the workings of these natural resources – our own endogenous drugs – so that we can create the conditions that will enable them to do

> what they do best, with minimal interferences from exogenous substances ... or to create ... drugs that imitate the natural substances and cause minimal interference with the bodymind's balance because they have been developed with an awareness of the whole psychosomatic network (Pert, 1997: 271-272).

Bloom (1997), a US psychiatrist, also describes this phenomenon of body memory in her writing on the mental health effects of trauma and abuse. She began asking patients about past experiences of trauma, and found that over 80 per cent recounted 'horrific stories of trauma of all kinds, which occurred usually in childhood' (Bloom, 1997: 109). Many had reported this at an initial history-taking exercise but staff had not acted on the information. Others had not told their story because they had not been asked. On discovering the extent of trauma, Bloom developed a hospital sanctuary in which people could safely reveal and deal with their traumas and recover from them.

> It became apparent to us that trauma does indeed do terrible things to the body's physiology ... we had to struggle with differentiating between pain associated with structural or functional physical problems and the pain associated with 'body memories' ... When a body memory occurs, the victim actually experiences pain, so his or her distress is quite real (Bloom, 1997: 156-157).

Bloom argues that the tragedy in people's lives can be transcended and transformed. The symptoms displayed by patients in mental health crisis are a clue to their personal tragedies, and a way of seeking the response they need to 'find a place back within the human community':

> it is this response that we had repeatedly [before the change to the sanctuary hospital] failed to give, creating instead a society that revolved around unconscious and repeated trauma, instead of change, transcendence, and transformation (Bloom, 1997: 193).

The work of Pert, Bloom and others who have looked at the mind/body/spirit connections in new ways, could help provide the scientific basis for transforming the biomedical model of mental illness to a no less evidence-based but more holistic and psychosocial discourse with the aim of ceasing to put blocks in the way of recovery and helping to promote healing and well-being.

Recovery and the Role of Service Providers

Our system makes it possible for people with mental health problems to adopt a 'sick role' but the transition back to social inclusion is often more difficult. The bureaucracy of services and benefits forces people to prove they are seriously disordered to qualify for help, and forces them through another set of hoops if they want to return to work. The lack of flexibility in the benefits system mirrors the social stigma attached to mental illness, displaying a lack of trust in the willingness of most people to make a contribution to society, as well as a failure to understand the invisible scars that make it hard for many who have experienced mental health problems to return seamlessly and without problems to full time paid work.

Good relationships between staff and service users help recovery, according to the British Psychological Society (BPS, 2000). The Psychosis Revisited training pack (BPS, 2003) calls for recognition of the power differentials between workers and service users, and points out the contradictory roles of care and control played by mental health services. They suggest that workers need regular supervision and emotional support to enable them to maintain a collaborative, less controlling approach with people having psychotic experiences.

Conclusion

The recovery concept can help to guide the planning and implementation of services and supports for people with severe mental illness. A recovery approach respects lived experience and expertise, and can contribute to the revitalisation of psychiatric science in line with the changes in other modern sciences towards understanding the actual complexity of human life in society and the natural environment. Ultimately, we all need to recover, from an era in which the abuse of women and children was kept hidden behind closed doors, from a past riven with class discrimination and racist oppression, from a work ethic that has made it hard for many people to have any quality of life. We need to heal communities where members feel lonely and isolated, where children, young people and older people are cut off from each other. We need to halt the disintegration of supportive communities, and promote an education system that engages children's creativity and enthusiasm and enables them to become active and responsible citizens, prepared for a rapidly changing world

References

Baker, S. and Strong, S. (2001), 'Roads to Recovery: How people with mental health problems recover and find ways of coping', Mind, www.mind.org.uk.

Beresford, P. and Hopton, J. (2003), 'Recovery or independent living?', *Openmind* 124, November/December, 16-17.

Bloom, S. (1997), *Creating Sanctuary: Towards the Evolution of Sane Societies*, New York: Routledge.

Boyle, M. (1996), 'Schizophrenia: The fallacy of diagnosis', *Changes*, **14**(1), 5-13.

The British Psychological Society, Division of Clinical Psychology (2000), *Recent advances in understanding mental illness and psychotic experiences report*, Leicester: The British Psychological Society.

The British Psychological Society, Division of Clinical Psychology (2003), *The Psychosis Revisited Training Pack*, Leicester: The British Psychological Society.

Capra, F. (1983), *The Turning Point*, London: Flamingo.

Ciompi, L. (1980), 'Lausanne studies', in the *Schizophrenia Bulletin*, 6, 606-618.

Copeland, M.E. (1997), *Wellness Recovery Action*, in Brattleboro, VT: Peach Press.

Deegan, P. (2001), Recovery as a Self-Directed Process of Healing and Transformation, www.intentionalcare.org/articles/articles_trans.pdf.

Desisto, M.J., Harding, C.M., McCormick, R.V., Ashikaga, T. and Brooks, G.W. (1995), The Maine and Vermont three-decade studies of serious mental illness, I and II, *The British Journal of Psychiatry*, 161, 331-342.

Faulkner, A. and Layzell, S. (2000), *Strategies for Living: A report of user-led research into people's strategies for living with mental distress*, London: Mental Health Foundation.

Grof, S. and Grof, C. (eds) (1989), *Spiritual emergency: When Personal Transformation Becomes a Crisis*, New York: G.P. Putnam's Sons.

Huber, G., Gross, G., Schuttler, R. and Linz, M. (1980), 'Longtitudinal studies of schizophrenic patients', *Schizophrenia Bulletin*, 6(4), 592-605.

Johnson, S., Ramsey, R., Thornicroft, G., Brooks, L., Lelliott, P., Peck, E., Smith, H., Chisholm, D., Audini, B., Knapp, M. and Goldberg, D. (eds) (1997), *London's Mental Health: The report to the King's Fund London Commission*, London: Kings Fund.

Kruger, A. (2000), 'Schizophrenia: Recovery and hope', *Psychiatric Rehabilitation Journal*, 24(1), 29-37.

Levinson, R., Greatley, A. and Robinson, J. (2003), *London's State of Mind: Kings Fund mental health inquiry 2003*, London: Kings Fund.

MDF, *Inside Out – An Introduction to Self Management*, Manic Depression Fellowship booklet.

Mental Health Commission (2001), *Mental Health Recovery Competencies Teaching Resource Kit*, New Zealand: Mental Health Commission. Email: info@mhc.govt.nz.

McLean, A. (2003), 'Recovering Consumers and a Broken Mental Health System in the United States: Ongoing Challenges for Consumers/Survivors and the New Freedom Commission on Mental Health', *International Journal of Psychosocial Rehabilitation*, 8, 47-68.

Michaelson, J. and Wallcraft, J. (1997), 'Alternatives to the biomedical model of mental health crisis', *Breakthrough* 1(3), 31-49.

NAMI (Santa Cruz County) (2004), www.namiscc.org/Recovery.

NSF (2001), Recovery in NSF (available as a pdf file on www.rethink.org/recovery/).

Ogawa, K. *et al.* (1987), 'Japanese studies', in *The British Journal of Psychiatry*, 151, 678-765.

Onken, S.J., Dumont, J.M., Ridgway, P., Dornan, D.H. and Ralph, R.O. (2002), *Phase One Research Report: A National Study of Consumer Perspectives on What Helps and Hinders Mental Health Recovery*, National Association of State Mental Health Program Directors (NASMHPD) National Technical Assistance Center (NTAC), Alexandria: VA.

Pert, C. (1998), *Molecules of Emotion: Why You Feel the Say You Feel*, Simon and Schuster Ltd.

Popper, K. (1987), *The Logic of Scientific Discovery*, London: Hutchinson.

Repper, J. and Perkins R. (2003), *Social Inclusion and Recovery*, London, Balliere Tindall.

Rethink (2004), webpage on recovery www.rethink.org/recovery/.

SCMH (1998), *Acute Problems: A Survey of the Quality of Care in Acute Psychiatric Wards*, London: Sainsbury Centre for Mental Health.

Secker, J. (2004), 'All Shook Up: What Mental Health Research Means to Me', *The Mental Health Review* 9(1), March 2004, 32-40.

S.H.A.R.P. (2001), Mid-Term Review, Supported Housing and Recovery Project, Hereford (unpublished paper).

Thornton, L. (2004), Recovery From Schizophrenia, www.namiscc.org/.

Torrey, E.F. and Zdanowicz, M. (2001), Outpatient commitment: What, why, and for whom, *Psychiatric Services*, 52, 337-341.

Chapter 10

Self-Help/Mutual Aid as a Psychosocial Phenomenon

Carol Munn-Giddings and Thomasina Borkman

In the introductory chapter to this book Ramon and Williams suggest that a paradigm shift is beginning in the field of mental health, what they call 'psychosocial' of which there will be a plurality of versions. In this chapter we offer a model of self-help/mutual aid groups focusing on persons with mental health problems who autonomously run them. We suggest that experienced self-helpers and self-help/mutual aid groups that have developed experiential knowledge of living with mental health problems and navigating the mental health and social services systems embody a psychosocial approach to mental health problems that is holistic, person-centred, contextual, and integrates the psychological, social, and biological.

Drawing primarily on the literature from our reciprocal countries, the UK and USA, we provide an overview of the distinguishing features of self-help/mutual aid groups and explore the nature of the collective knowledge built over time by peers who share their direct experiences and the potential challenge this poses to the existing medical model of mental health. Throughout the chapter we highlight the unique support that people can gain from self-help/mutual aid groups, whilst providing example(s) of the innovation in practice that can occur when mental health practitioners work alongside people with direct experience of mental health problems. Finally we suggest an emerging approach developing from our cross-cultural research with self-help/mutual aid groups that focuses on self-directed 'recovery' with the assistance of experiential peers (Borkman *et al.*, 2004).

Context

Mutual support and voluntary action have always been a part of human societies; but, it is only since the 1970s that single issue self-help/mutual aid groups have been observed and documented across Europe, North America, Japan, Australia and New Zealand (Borkman, 1999; Hastie, 2000; Munn-Giddings, 2003). Self-help/mutual aid groups have formed the backbone of the mental health service user movement in both the UK and North America and are cited as a significant component of peer-orientated and led initiatives in these other countries (Everett, 1994; Wallcraft and Bryant, 2003). Underlying the movements has been the collective concern to change both traditional mental health services and broader societal attitudes.

However, it is from the 1970s in UK and the USA that groups explicitly critical of psychiatry began to emerge raising awareness about issues such as conditions on psychiatric wards, closures of long-stay hospitals and matters affecting their quality of life. Wallcraft and Bryant (2003) note that in UK patient only groups such as the Mental Patients Union and the Campaign Against Psychiatric Oppression (CAPO formerly COPE) emerged at this time alongside pressure group organisations (not led by service users) such as MIND and the National Schizophrenic Fellowship (now Rethink). Some alliances were also being formed between patients and professionals such as Survivors Speak Out (SSO). In North America extensive diversity was found in the ideologies of groups and their relationships with mental health professionals and the mental health system. Radical groups such as 'Mad Liberation' distanced themselves from professionals and the system feeling they had been victimised by it whilst others such as Recovery Inc (initially founded in 1937 by the psychiatrist Abraham Low) had groups willing to work with professionals. Everett (1994) viewed the loose network of groups as an important social movement distinguishable because service users rather than professionals or philanthropists led it.

However it was in the 1980s in the UK that there was a major increase in patients councils, self-help groups and user forums (the latter of which were often instigated by professionals specifically to influence local services). The model for both groups and councils were heavily influenced by the Dutch Patients Councils and US User Movement which underlined the importance of mutual support and consciousness-raising. Wallcraft and Bryant (2003) state that four significant UK user networks with associated self-help groups were formed in this time: UK Advocacy Network (UKAN), Survivors Speak Out (SSO); National Voices Network (NVN) and the Hearing Voices Network all to provide support, share information, campaign for change and challenge discrimination.

Brandon (1991) and Lindlow (1994) also describe a number of grassroots self-help groups from specific localities in a number of countries, such as Womankind set up in Bristol, England in 1985 to promote mental health in women. Womankind was a multi-racial project that enabled over 50 women to meet monthly and share experiences. They organised a conference of 100 women who specifically addressed from their own experience what helped and hindered them in the psychiatric system.

Brandon notes that a distinctive feature of UK groups is that few have taken a separatist line and have tended to work towards partnership and co-operation with progressive professionals, citing a number of examples of this work (1991: 154-5). Lindlow (1994) concurs with this view although raises concerns about the possible co-option of service users by the system. By contrast, the US service movement has from early days emphasised self-help alternatives to existing services. Although as Chamberlin (1990) notes, as self-help alternatives proliferated the radical voices within the US movement tended to weaken.

What is stunning about these movements is that they turned the conventional way of thinking about reform on its head. Instead of the stereotypical view of sick and dependent persons, people with mental health problems are seen as active agents who not only forcefully demand choices in their treatment, but also want to be involved in its design, implementation and evaluation. In the UK government policy both enabled and responded to these demands to some extent by mandating that service users must be involved in services; the extent to which the policy has been substantively implemented is another question. US policy has shifted much less dramatically; incorporating people with mental health problems into policy making and involvement in services is quite limited. However in both countries self-help/mutual aid groups and networks working with other activists have achieved a number of successes. Chamberlin emphasises that in the US people with mental health problems are represented in forums and legislative hearings, engaged in advocacy to end involuntary treatment and have developed self-help programmes as alternatives to professional treatment (Chamberlin, 1990).

Despite the inevitable cultural differences between the mental health movements in different countries important common features can be discerned:

- The central importance of self-help/mutual aid groups
- The central importance of mutual support
- Sharing of experiences, information and coping strategies
- Protest against traditional service provision
- Recognition that people may need temporary or ongoing support
- Championing the importance of choice and freedom
- Advocating groups and services that are service user centred or controlled.

Self-help/mutual aids groups clearly then have a role to play in a psychosocial model of mental health care. In the next section we look at some of the unique features of groups, their processes and benefits comparing them to traditional medical model services.

What are Self-help/Mutual Aid Groups?

Although there is no single agreed upon definition of self-help/mutual aid groups, there is consensus among researchers of at least three commonalities:

- They are run for and by people who share the same health or social issue
- Their primary source of knowledge is based on sharing direct experience
- They occur as voluntary collectives predominantly in the third sector of society as opposed to the statutory or private sectors.

We distinguish groups from 'self-help' on an individual level which is often associated with the personal use of a range of books, audio-tapes, video-tapes and T.V. programmes that are specifically intended to provide individuals with useful information and suggested 'coping strategies'. Self-help on an individual level also frequently refers to an individual taking responsibility for problem solving his/her troubles while mutual aid refers to the context of one's relationship with peers who give to and support each other. We deliberately combine the terms (self-help/mutual aid) because we believe that it is the combination of self-responsibility with the reciprocity (mutuality) of relationship with others and the consequent processes within the groups that enables the individuals to help themselves.

Forms of self-help vary greatly, from face-to-face groups (of many types and sizes) and telephone helplines to, increasingly, 'virtual' mutual aid using (Web-based) discussion boards, chatrooms, e-mail groups and lists such as Borderline UK.

Because groups are based on the principle of peer 'reciprocity', the relationships are quite different to those in traditional services where a 'user', 'client' or 'patient' is dependent on the advice, support or treatment of a professional. Ownership and power are the crucial factors distinguishing the professionally led group (often known as 'support groups') and the self-help/mutual aid group. Ownership for the self-helper arises from the sharing of personal experience and the experiential knowledge generated from such activity within a context where peers lead and control their own group. Even when practitioners share this same experience or perspective, the most sympathetic practitioners are likely to have a vested and powerful interest in maintaining a professional discourse and knowledge base.

In North America many self-help groups are based on the 12-step programme established by Alcoholics Anonymous (AA). In the USA over 100 12-step groups for conditions other than alcoholism have been established (White and Madara, 2002); and it is estimated that one third of self-help groups in the USA are 12-step groups (Wuthnow, 1994). A great deal of the US literature is based on studies of these groups, and the 12-step groups are so well known that they are an integral part of US popular culture (Room, 1992). In the UK, however, it would appear from the available and recent literature (Elsdon *et al.*, 2000) that very few groups follow this model. They are not well known or understood in the UK culture.

It is notable that although there is considerable research interest in the service user movement, self-help/mutual aid groups themselves are under-researched in the UK (Elsdon *et al.*, 2000; Munn-Giddings, 2003; Wright, 2004) and in the main the dominant literature comes from the USA, chiefly from the disciplines of psychology and social work which tend to understand and frame self-help/mutual aid groups in relation to therapeutic groups or human/social services, such as Katz and Bender (1976) and Riessman (1990). Humphreys and Rappaport (1994) and Borkman (1999) point out that this is problematic since groups are then only rarely viewed in the context of their role in the broader society. However some studies are exploring self-help/mutual aid groups alongside other social support networks such as faith groups, and citizen action groups (Antze, 1976; Kurtz and Powell, 1987; Messer and Borkman, 1996) or placing self-help/mutual aid groups within a 'political action' framework (Chamberlin and Rogers, 1990; Maton, 1993). These frameworks are concerned with the evolution of campaigning or advocacy groups that emphasise the location of the shared problems in the wider cultures of society, such as the women's movement, disability movements and gay rights movements. They share an interest not only in personal changes but also how group processes can affect the groups' views and perspectives on their situations. Borkman (1999) has more recently termed her own approach as a 'voluntary action' one stressing the voluntary nature of these groups, viewed as occupying an important part of the third sector of society. The perspectives, with which researchers have conceptualised self-help/mutual aid groups, clearly have an impact on the type of study carried out and the benefits and effects attributed to group membership.

In both the UK and the USA, it has been very difficult to map and document self-help/mutual aid activity because of its fluid and informal nature as well as the lack of researcher and policy interest. There are no national databases that list a census of self-help groups in the UK or USA. In the US the American Self-Help Clearinghouse, a national level resource centre, has an online database and a hard copy directory of national and model groups (White and Madara, 2002) but not of local groups. However, long term observers, some local/regional studies (Elsdon *et al.*, 2000) and the increased size of directories over time provide overwhelming anecdotal evidence that the number and type of groups has been increasing.

The estimate in Elsdon and colleagues' recent study (2000) is that there are approximately 23,400 health related self-help groups in the UK and that four per cent of the adult population are likely to belong to a self-help group. Wuthnow (1994) estimated that in the USA eight to ten million adults belonged to approximately 500,000 self-help groups which is also about four per cent of the adult population who are likely to belong to a group. In addition to having little trustworthy information about the number of groups or the number of people attending them, the demographic characteristics of members is not reliably known. Perhaps the most trustworthy estimate is that both in the USA and UK more women attend most groups than men (Wann, 1995; Kurtz, 1997). Statistics on age, race/ethnicity or socio-economic status are so local or unrepresentative as to be misleading and better left unreported.

Whilst we do not have any comprehensive map of mental health self-help/mutual aid groups in the UK we have some indication of size from Wallcraft and Bryant's (2003) study of the service user movement in the UK. Their survey had responses from 318 local groups across the country with a membership of over 9,000 people. They identified six national service user/survivor networks of 6,800 individuals and 450 local affiliated groups. They noted that United Kingdom Advocacy Network (UKAN) has over 300 groups affiliated, and the Hearing Voices Network has 150 local groups. Also apparent from their survey is that women are generally reasonably well represented in groups (although this varies) and that minority ethnic groups are not well represented. It is also important to recognise that self-help groups on the Internet are blossoming and may offer a more anonymous source of support with the UK Depression Alliance website, for instance, claiming to receive over 500,000 page views every month (Depression Alliance, 2000).

This trend toward an increasing number of self-help groups is replicated in Scandinavia and other parts of Europe (Hastie, 2000; Nylund, 2000; Karlsson, 2000). Groups are also developing in post-communist countries. In Hungary alone, some 30,000 voluntary organisations including 2,000 to 3,000 self-help groups had registered by 1993.

Experiential Knowledge

Probably the core process in all self-help/mutual aid groups is the sharing of personal experience through telling stories about living with the focal issue, what Borkman in 1976 termed 'experiential knowledge': 'Experiential knowledge is truth learned from personal experience with a phenomenon rather than truth acquired by discursive reasoning, observation or reflection on information provided by others ... it is subjectively based' (Borkman, 1976: 446). Professional and scientific knowledge have predominated as the legitimate source of information and wisdom in this era. However, the social movements of the 1970s and later civil rights of minority groups – the women's movement, the disability rights movement, among others – have championed the importance of experiential knowledge as a distinctive and important source of knowledge. Borkman (1990) suggested that the importance of this knowledge is underestimated especially in policy and service developments; she views the collective knowledge built over time in a group as critically affecting the group's and thus its members' potential to reconceptualise the issues they face and often to go beyond the narrow technical or scientific framework that physicians and other professionals have given them. It is

> 'subjectively based' knowledge that integrates the feelings, thoughts and ideas about the experience ... a reflective process is necessary to convert 'raw experience', which is often a jumble of inchoate images, thoughts, impressions and feelings, into knowledge (which implies some form, coherence and meaning). The reflective process can be done by oneself or with others, as when one talks about one's experience. A key point about self-help groups is that the reflective process is done with others who have shared the same experience and thus have specialised knowledge about it and a personal stake in its interpretation (Borkman, 1990: 15-16).

Individuals who listen to their peers' stories learn, among other things, what about their experience of living with the focal problem is unique (often because of their total life context), and what is common to many of their peers. They thus learn more generally the forms, contours, and variety of issues that people with their problem live with and they can put their own idiosyncratic experience into this larger context. Individuals who do not share their direct experience with others may 'know' about their own experience but do not know the limits of their experience, that is, to what extent it can be generalised or applies to others like themselves. The difference between individual and collective knowledge that has been developed over time is largely unrecognised in policy and service developments.

This communal learning can produce what Borkman terms 'disciplined subjectivity', which is qualitatively different from one person's idiosyncratic interpretation of their own experience: ... the definition includes the sense that the person has some conviction that the experience he/she has reflected upon and processed is in fact knowledge and understanding (Borkman, 1999: 16).

An important aspect of knowledge held, distilled and shared in a self-help/mutual aid group is that it will become part of the collective knowledge, passed on even when the initiators leave the group.

The mode in which self-help/mutual aid groups communicate their experiential knowledge and perspective is by telling their stories; this has been noted and illustrated by many self-help/mutual aid researchers (Cain, 1991; Humphreys, 1992; Rappaport, 1993). This process in self-help/mutual aid can be contrasted with the formal dialogue in professions. Professional encounters often decontextualise 'information' about one's health or social situation whereas experiential knowledge is utterly contextualised. Brody (1987) argued that medical personnel devalue personal narratives by expecting patients to restrict their medical history to a litany of symptoms.

Rappaport (2000) discusses the importance to both individual and social change of building and recasting a shared narrative in ways that challenge dominant stereotypes conveyed through the mass media and other social and cultural institutions. Using GROW (a 12-step group founded in Australia by people with mental health problems) as one example, he explores how an individual's identity is constructed through the appropriation of a shared narrative into one's personal life story. Where someone with mental health problems is able to tell their own story and listen to others peers expressing theirs they may recast their experience. Citing Kloos (1999) comparative study of GROW members with mainstream service users, Rappaport notes how members of GROW had developed a shared 'normative community narrative' which influenced how their members understood themselves, thought about their future and developed a sense of personal identity. GROW members, who had many examples from their peers who had 'recovered' and were leading active lives in the community defined their lives in quite different ways from the users of mainstream services. For example, they defined their goals as self-development and creating a sense of community, whilst people using mainstream services prioritised taking medication and getting out on their own. GROW members continued to use medication but not see it as central to their self-definition. As Kennedy and Humphreys (1994) state belief systems or worldviews are at the core of mutual help because self-help groups are communities of belief not programmes of treatment or coping. People who join and stay in a group are likely to begin to assimilate its story into their own.

In the broader therapeutic literature it is recognised both cognitively and emotionally that re-telling your story is important (Bisbey and Bisbey, 1998). The potential to reframe experience(s) through repetition comes both from hearing others perspectives and hearing/examining your own voice. The distinctions in self-help/mutual groups being that the other voices are peers. Munn-Giddings (2003) has noted the subtle processes involved in some self-help groups where the juxtaposing of different individual stories about a similar issue enables members to broaden their perspectives on their own and others experience.

The importance of long-standing groups and membership becomes important in this context. Self-help groups vary in their organisational characteristics including their degree of formalisation and their longevity. Newer or fledgling groups are unlikely to have developed a self-empowering 'meaning perspective' (Borkman, 1999) or 'normative community narrative' (Rappaport, 2000) about their problem and their unseasoned members are uncertain and unlikely to have confidence in their lived experience of mental health problems. Developed groups have communicated enough about their personal experiences to have built a body of experiential knowledge and subsequently their seasoned members have confidence in and exert authority of their experiential knowledge of mental health problems (Borkman, 1999). Developed groups can distinguish between professional knowledge that is valuable and helpful and that which needs to be challenged, adapted or rejected. In contrast, fledgling groups lack enough experiential knowledge to discern helpful from unhelpful professional knowledge and may accept or reject it uncritically.

These processes underline the distinction between individual self-help and collective self-help. The reciprocal sharing of stories involved in groups is not only a feature of group relations but also can be seen as an important part of the group process that builds the trust enabling active members to exchange their stories and experiences. The form that reciprocity takes in grassroots self-help/mutual aid groups can primarily be seen as two-fold. Firstly, because membership is voluntary, active members engage in a series of freely given 'exchanges' of stories, support, advice and so on; the process is therefore one of a pattern of reciprocal exchanges. Active members are in the position of both giving and receiving support and advice. Much of the US literature refers to these exchanges as the 'gift' culture of self-help/mutual aid groups.

Secondly, some studies of self-help/mutual aid groups suggest that the reciprocity in groups is not always 'direct' but rather entails what is termed 'serial reciprocity'. This is where a new member receives support and advice from her peers but 'repays' this at a later stage in her own development by reciprocating the support either to her established peers or to a new member of the group (Katz and Bender, 1976; Gartner and Riessman, 1977; Richardson and Goodman, 1983).

Not surprisingly therefore active membership of a self-help/mutual aid group can lead to a number of benefits at both the individual and collective level.

Individual and Group Gains

A number of empirical studies in various health and social care areas, including mental health, have found that attendance at a self-help/mutual aid group leads to an improvement and/or management in aspects of the condition or situation. Table 10.1 summarises commonly attributed benefits from attending groups. These benefits are drawn from studies on a wide spectrum of self-help/mutual aid groups, using a variety of methodologies; each study may have focused on personal, interpersonal or collective gains but the Table lists any gain that was found in an individual study.

Table 10.1 Benefits derived from attending self-help/mutual aid groups

PERSONAL	INTER-PERSONAL	COLLECTIVE
improved self-esteem	mutual support	broader world view
improved self-confidence	mutual sharing of experience	collective perspective and mobilisation for social change or service innovation
improved emotional well-being	comradeship	opportunity to influence services
practical information	friendship	critiques of professional practices
practical support	not feeling alone	innovative relations w/mental health system
emotional support	sharing coping mechanisms	alternative ways to get help
feeling less isolated		deconstruction/critique of medical diagnoses or condition
feeling accepted		
spirituality		
learning new skills		

This table is expanded from a version found in Backwith and Munn-Giddings (2003) and draws on research from: Charlton and Barrow, 2002; Denzin, 1987; Elsdon et al., 2000; Faulkner and Layzell, 2000; Humphreys and Rappaport, 1994; Kurtz, 1997; Markowitz, 2001; Medvene, 1990; Munn-Giddings, 2003; Smith and Clarke, 2003; Suler, 1984; Thoburn, 1987; Trojan, 1989; Wann, 1995; Wilson, 1995.

Reviews of mental health specific studies resonate with the above features and add some additional outcomes. For example, Hatzidimitriadou's study (2002) of 14 mental health self-help/mutual aid groups in England examined the role of political ideology and the psychosocial characteristics of group members. The findings suggested that whilst groups shared limited social networks and supports and marginal well-being group members felt empowered and experienced a number of helping processes. It was noted that more radical groups reported a sense of optimism and control over their lives, less radical groups benefiting primarily from sharing feelings and self-disclosure. Kyrouz and Humphreys (2004) review included studies which compared mental health episodes and admissions to hospital between those who do and do not attend groups, there was a consistent finding that active group membership resulted in reducing members' use of services.

Importantly, many of these types of features have been reinforced by recent research from the user-led research team 'Strategies for Living' based at the

Mental Health Foundation in the UK. Wright (2004) notes that in the six years of supporting user-led research (which has involved 40 researchers in more than 20 projects) a consistent finding has been the importance attributed to self-help, mutual support and shared experience: 'Service users and people who experience mental distress share the desire to meet with other people who have similar experiences to share information, share coping strategies, feel accepted and included and form relationships' (Wright, 2004: 2). Similarly, the recent survey of mental health user groups by the Sainsbury Centre found that user groups accorded most priority to self-help and social support (Wallcraft and Bryant, 2003). A recent study by service users (Smith and Clarke, 2003) of nine self-groups for people who self-harm found that two-thirds of participants (n=34) stated that they felt accepted, valued and not-judged as a result of attending the group. Two-thirds also had experienced a reduction in isolation and cited making friends as an important result of group attendance. Helping others was also an important theme to emerge which members felt had boosted their self-esteem as it highlighted their strengths and abilities. All but two of those interviewed felt group membership had a positive aspect on their emotional and mental well-being.

A drawback to self-help/mutual aid groups is that they may suit or benefit only a small percentage of eligible members (Kaufmann *et al.*, 1994). However, the features outlined above hold for many the potential to regain or gain some control back over their lives with supportive peers, especially those actively involved over a long period of time. Many of the features such as feeling accepted, building new friendships and skills can be important aspects in countering social exclusion and isolation often associated with mental distress (Dunn, 1999). As Wright states 'self-help groups provide support for individuals when possibly there is no other support available OR provide the only support which feels accepting and empowering' (2004: 3).

Messer and Borkman (1996) have argued that the types of skills members acquire in groups, such as organisational skills, understanding others' perspectives and comradeship, are building a form of 'social capital' in the community that can be translated into other areas. Elsdon *et al.* (2000) in the UK have made a similar point: defining the types of learning that go on in-group as related to content (about the issues being faced), social and personal learning (such as self-knowledge, social skills) and political learning (managing problems of authority and conflict). They view the latter as developing leadership skills that could transcend the group setting.

Experiential Knowledge and Professionals

We are not claiming that self-help/mutual aid groups are a substitute for services rather that they offer unique features and relations that cannot be replicated by professional-user relations. However there are likely to be tensions between professionals who adhere to a medical model of mental health and self-help/mutual aid groups. Professionals may not alert service users to relevant groups as they fear 'misinformation' or increased emotional distress resulting from attendance (Wann,

1995). Wilson (1995) pointed out that professionals and self-help/mutual aid groups inhabit two very different worlds. Self-help/mutual aid groups provide important services that can complement or challenge those traditionally offered by human service organisations. Yet for ideological and structural reasons there is a tension between self-help groups and services, which may evolve under certain conditions towards either conflict or co-operation.

> The nature of professionalism endorses the professional as expert, using knowledge refined through long years of practice and gained through training. The self-helper uses experiential knowledge, and has expertise from living with a problem. Professionals, who seriously want to work with self-help groups will have to reappraise their own roles, accept the strengths and potential strengths of their clients and be prepared to give up some of their power (Wilson, 1995: 58).

Wilson's UK study of 49 diverse groups and 50 professionals concluded that professionals found it difficult to perceive groups as anything other than an adjunct to professional services. They assumed, for example, that people joined groups in order to influence services, whereas members' primary concern was mutual support and information. The importance that members attributed to giving as well as receiving support was also underestimated. More recently Elsdon *et al.* (2000) have come to similar conclusions.

Similarly, in the USA Salzer *et al.* (2001) surveyed 895 mental health professionals to assess the differences in their attitudes and behaviours towards professionally-led and peer-led groups. An important finding was that professionals who perceived professionally led groups to be more significant than peer groups were unlikely to support peer groups through referrals and finance. The study concluded that professionals need to be more aware of the role and benefits that peer self-help groups can contribute to expanding the availability and continuum of beneficial mental health services (Salzer in Wright, 2004).

However, whilst we have pointed out the differences between support systems based on experiential peer relations and traditional medical model services it is also important to acknowledge and celebrate the partnerships that have occurred between professionals who are committed to exploring the different understandings that service users have to offer.

A good example of this is the work of Professor Romme, a Dutch Psychiatrist from the University of Limburg, whose openness to listening to the alternative ways of coping suggested by service users who heard voices poses a challenge to the traditional medical model on two counts. The story begins in the mid 1980s with Romme being surprised by a woman service user whose medication to alleviate her (threatening) voices was not working but who gained comfort from knowing that others heard voices and that in ancient times this was considered 'normal practice'. Romme's willingness to move outside the medical model and explore with other service users their experiences led him to meet and discuss these issues in small groups and via a TV broadcast gain the views of another 700 service users on their experience of voices and their coping mechanisms. Along with Escher (a journalist) Romme's research into the area (based on the issues raised by service users) led to some challenging findings (Romme and Escher, 1993). Key amongst these were that:

- Many people in the general population both hear and cope with voices and as such hearing voices in itself is not necessarily evidence of a 'psychotic illness'
- Whilst some service users consider their voices threatening many consider them beneficial
- Service users are aware that the voices do not indicate the presence of a real person, even if they represent one
- Living with voices has led service users to develop useful coping mechanisms which can usefully be shared with others in the same situation.

Combined these findings have led to the development of the Dutch and British Hearing Voices Network (HVN), a loose network of self-help/mutual aid groups for people who hear voices. The HVN has both symbolically and literally challenged the traditional service intervention of suppressing voices through medication by providing an alternative way for peers to support one another. Other examples of professional-service user alliances are also encouraging (Castillo *et al.*, 2001).

**Table 10.2   Differences in the experiential and medical models of mental
            health**

	Experiential Model	**Medical Model**
Type of Organisation	Informal	Formal
Form of Relationships	Peer	Hierarchical
Type of Relationship	Reciprocal	Dependent
Form of Attendance	Participatory	Passive
Type of Attendance	Voluntary	Voluntary-Compulsory
Type of Knowledge	Theory from direct individual and collective experience	Theory from abstract and indirect professional experience
Exchange of knowledge:	Sharing stories	Professional elicits symptoms from service user and controls the interaction
	Contexualised	Decontexualised
	Holistic	Compartmentalised
Type of benefit	Intra-personal/Collective	Individual

Interestingly Hodges *et al.*, recent study (2003) suggests that mental health self-helpers are deriving a greater satisfaction from mainstream services because they are able to make more appropriate use of them. Therefore self-helpers are more likely to be discerning, assertive users of mainstream services, which does not diminish the need of services but suggests it will lead to a change in the nature of service use. Hence there is some optimism for the potential of professionally led services to complement self-help/mutual aid activities. However on a range of indicators it is clear from the above discussion that there are major differences between the medical model and experiential model of care and support as illustrated in Table 10.2.

Towards an Evolving Approach: From Community Service Recipient to Recovering Citizen

From the above discussion we wish to reinforce the significance of both experiential knowledge and the collective processes that self-helpers go through in relation to core strands of the psychosocial model. Our study of mental health self-help/mutual aid groups emphasises the active agency and capability of the person with mental health problems. This resonates with the bold claims and approaches advocated for many years by 'Mad Liberation', the service user movement and sympathetic professionals including ex-patients with professional roles (Beresford, 1997; Brandon, 1991; Campbell, 1987; Croft and Beresford, 1993; Ramon, 1996).

In both the USA and the UK in the professional services the possibility that people with even severe mental illness can 'recover' and regain or construct a meaningful life as citizens is gaining currency. Many professional clinicians as well as policy analysts are now interested in the concept of recovery (Anthony 2000; Carpenter 2002; Department of Health, 2001). The concept of recovery is well known in the USA and Canada (Room, 1992), but less so in the UK. In the USA it is drawn from the experience of Alcoholics Anonymous (AA) a 12-step self-help/mutual aid group controlled by its members who identify themselves as recovering alcoholics and without any professionals. Hundreds of thousands of AA members have stopped drinking alcohol and developed or resumed constructive work, family, and community lives. In the addictions area, recovery is understood to be a self-directed process of gaining a constructive and positive way of living within a context of mutual aid and support from experiential peers; assistance from professionals is also sought sometimes. Some mental health professionals think that recovery as a primarily self and peer directed process can be applied to mental health problems but with some differences. Unlike thousands of alcoholics and drug addicts who recovered primarily with the aid of self-help groups and outside of professional services and without pharmacological intervention, severe mental illness is much more likely to involve the expertise of psychiatrists and pharmacological intervention and to involve recurring symptoms.

In the UK, as Wallcraft has outlined in Tew (2004), the notion of recovery is mainly attributed to service users own narratives of recovery. In addition empirical studies have illuminated the importance of social and psychological factors such as employment, housing, social support and friendships that are as crucial as psychiatric interventions in enabling people with mental health problems to construct and retain a meaningful life in their community (Faulkner and Layzell, 2000; Turner-Crowson and Wallcraft, 2002). The UK literature stresses the importance of service users defining their own vision of 'recovery', it is not necessary for people to define (or accept) themselves as mentally ill but it is important to recognise and explore one's problems.

Although the origins of the concept of recovery can be seen to differ between countries, the central aspect of regaining or taking control of one's own life is common. In both the importance of supportive relationships particularly with experientially knowledgeable peers is also central yet under-recognised by professional services. Thus, the potential importance of self-help/mutual aid in the recovery process needs to be highlighted.

The emerging recovery approach also has implications at a systems level. The current dominant service approach focuses on the system of mental health services *as* controlled by professionals rather than service users and is based on the assumptions that the professional is the expert, in control, and is required to provide services to people with mental illness. In this model, people with mental illness are consulted about their preferences but the professional expert still maintains control. People with mental illness are physically present in the community but in segregated facilities and are not integrated as a valuable participant in the community.

In the new model (Anthony, 2000; Carpenter, 2002; Nelson *et al.*, 2001) the vision that people can recover from mental illness requires that the service delivery system must be redesigned to facilitate recovery. The stakeholders – the people with mental illness and their families – must have a major voice in designing, choosing, and utilising services with the expert role modified to 'support facilitator'. Stakeholders share power with the professional. Other key ideas are that recovery can occur without professional intervention (in fact a diagnosis from a professional is not even necessary for recovery to begin), even when symptoms reoccur. But the individual with mental health problems needs a network of positive support, especially self-help/mutual aid groups of peers, and choices of treatments, work and living arrangements (Borkman *et al.*, 2004). Persons with mental health problems are viewed as autonomous citizens with the same rights to quality housing, educational and job opportunities, and other roles as a valued and integral part of the community as other citizens.

Conclusion

We are arguing in this chapter that a pre-eminent version of a psychosocial approach is manifested and embodied by mental health members of a self-help/mutual aid group and their collectivity. The self-help/mutual aid group, a learning community that respects, values, accumulates and utilises the experiential knowledge and wisdom of its members, is also a powerful support mechanism to assist individuals, with the reciprocal help of their peers, to recover a constructive and positive life despite the recurrence of symptoms. The mental health self-helper and self-help/mutual aid group contribute a distinctive perspective and body of knowledge that differs from, challenges but may also complement professional knowledge about mental health.

References

Anthony, W. (2000), 'A recovery-oriented service system: Setting some system level Standards', *Psychiatric Rehabilitation Journal* **24**(2), 159-168.

Antze, P. (1976), 'The role of ideologies in peer psychotherapy groups', *Journal of Applied Behavioral Science*, **12**, 323-346.

Backwith, D. and Munn-Giddings, C. (2003), 'Self-help/mutual aid in promoting mental health at work', *Journal of Mental Health Promotion*, **2**(4): 14-25.

Beresford, P. (1997), 'New Movements, New Politics: Making Participation Possible', in Jordan, T. and Lent, A. (eds), *Storming the Millennium: The New Politics of Change*, London: Lawrence and Wishart.

Bisbey, S. and Bisbey, L. (1998), *Brief Therapy for PSTD: Traumatic Reduction and Related Techniques*, Chichester: John Wiley & Sons.

Borkman, T. (1976), 'Experiential knowledge: A new concept for the analysis of self-help groups', *Social Services Review*, **50**, 445-456.

Borkman, T. (1990), 'Experiential, Professional and Lay Frames of Reference', in Powell, T. (ed.), *Working with Self-Help*. Silver Spring, Md.: National Association of Social Workers.

Borkman, T. (1999), *Understanding Self-Help/Mutual Aid: Experiential Learning in the Commons*, New Brunswick: Rutgers University Press.

Borkman, T., Karlsson, M., Munn-Giddings, C. and Smith, L. (2004), *Cross-National Research with Mental Health Self-Help*, Stockholm, Sweden: Skondal Institute.

Brandon, D. (1991), *Innovation Without Change?: Consumer Power in Psychiatric Services*, Basingstoke: Macmillan Press.

Brody, H. (1987), *Stories of Sickness*, New Haven: Yale University Press.

Cain, C. (1991), 'Personal Stories: Identity Acquisition and Self-Understanding in Alcoholics Anonymous', *Ethos* **19**(2), 210-251.

Campbell, P. (1987), 'Giants and Goblins', in Baker, E. and Pecks, I. (eds), *Power in Strange Places: User Empowerment in Mental Health Services*, London: Good Practices in Mental Health.

Carpenter, J. (2002), 'Mental health recovery paradigm: Implications for social work', *Health and Social Work*, **27**(2), May, 86-94.

Castillo, H., Allen, L. and Coxhead, N. (2001), 'The hurtfulness of a diagnosis: User research about personality disorder', *Mental Health Practice*, **4**(9), 16-19.

Charlton, G. and Barrow, C. (2002), 'Coping and self-help group membership in Parkinson's disease: A qualitative study', *Health and Social Care in the Community*, **10**(6), 472-478.

Chamberlin, J. (1990), *On Our Own*, London: MIND.

Chamberlin, J. and Rogers, J.A. (1990), 'Planning a Community-based Mental Health System: Perspective of Service Recipients', *American Psychologist*, **45**, 1241-1244.

Croft, S. and Beresford, P. (1993), *Getting Involved: A Practical Manual*, London: Open Services Project.

Denzin, N.K. (1987), *The Recovering Alcoholic*, Newbury Park: Sage.

Department of Health (2001), *The Journey to Recovery – the Government's Vision for Mental Health Care*, London: The Stationery Office.

Depression Alliance (2000) Depression and work. *www.depressionalliance.org/ (accessed 19 November 2000).*

Dunn, S. (1999), *Creating Accepting Communities: Report of the MIND Inquiry into Social Exclusion and Mental Health Problems*, London: MIND.

Elsdon, K., Reynolds, J. and Stewart, S. (2000), *Sharing Experience, Living and Learning: A Study of Self-Help Groups*, London: Community Matters.

Everett, B. (1994), 'Something is happening: The contemporary consumer and psychiatric survivor movement in historical context', *Journal of Mind and Behaviour*, 15(1-2), 55-70.

Faulkner, A. and Layzell, S. (2000), *Strategies for Living: A report of user-led research into people's strategies for living with mental distress*, London: Mental Health Foundation.

Gartner, A. and Riessman, F. (1977), *Self-Help in the Human Services*, San Francisco: Jossey-Bass.

Hastie, N. (2000), 'International perspectives on self help', paper presented in *Framing a Future for Self Help*, Conference Report Derby, June: Nottingham: Self Help Nottingham.

Hatzidimitriadou, E. (2002), 'Political ideology, helping mechanisms and empowerment of mental health self-help/mutual aid groups', *Journal of Community and Applied Social Psychology*, 12(4), 271-285.

Hodges, J., Markward, M., Keele, C. and Evans, C. (2003), 'Use of Self-Help Services and Consumer Satisfaction with Professional Mental Health Services', *Psychiatric Services*, August 54, 1161-1163.

Humphreys, K. (1992), 'Twelve step stories and transformations in personal epistemology', in Community Narratives and Personal Stories symposium conducted at the meeting of the Midwestern Psychological Association.

Humphreys, K. and Rappaport, J. (1994), 'Researching self-help/mutual aid groups and organizations: Many roads, one journey', *Applied and Preventive Psychology*, 3, 217-231.

Karlsson, M. (2000), '*Self-Help Groups in Sweden*', paper presented at the International Society of Third Sector Research biennial conference, Dublin, July.

Katz, A.H. and Bender, E. (1976), *The Strength in US: Self Help Groups in the Modern World*, New York: Franklin-Watts.

Kaufmann, C., Schulberg, H. and Schooler, N. (1994), 'Self-help group participation among people with severe mental illness', *Prevention in Human Services*, 11(2), 315-331.

Kennedy, M. and Humphreys, K. (1994), 'Understanding worldview transformation in members of mutual help groups', *Prevention in Human Services*, 11(2), 181-198.

Kloos, B. (1999), 'Cultivating identity: Meaning-making in the context of residential treatment settings for persons with histories of psychological disorders', unpublished PhD dissertation, University of Illinois.

Kurtz, L.F., Powell, T.J. (1987), 'Three approaches to understanding self-help Groups', *Social Work with Groups*, b, 69-80.

Kurtz, L. (1997), Self-*Help and Support Groups: A Handbook for Practitioners*, Thousand Oaks, CA: Sage.

Kyrouz, E. and Humphreys, K. (2004), 'A review of research on the effectiveness of self-help mutual aid groups'. Mental Health Net, www.mentalhealth.net/articles/selfres.htm.

Lindlow, V. (1994), *Self-Help Alternatives to Mental Health Services*, London: MIND.

Markowitz, F. (2001), 'Modelling processes in recovery from mental illness: Relationships between symptoms, life satisfaction and self-concept', *Journal of Health and Social Behaviour*, 42(1), 64-79.

Maton, K.I. (1993), 'Moving beyond the individual level of analysis in mutual self-help group research: An ecological paradigm', *Journal of Applied Behavioral Science*, **29**, 272-286.

Medvene, L. (1990), *Selected Highlights of Research on Effectiveness of Self-Help Groups*, The California Self Help Center: UCLA.

Messer, J. and Borkman, T. (1996), 'Functions and Limits of Private and Public Benefit in Creating Social Capital: The Role of Self-Help Mutual Aid in Building Community Capacity', paper presented at the 25th annual conference of the Association for Research on Nonprofit Organizations and Voluntary Action: New York City, November.

Munn-Giddings, C. (2003), 'Mutuality and movement: An exploration of the relationship between self-help/mutual aid and social policy', unpublished doctoral thesis: Loughborough University.

Nelson, G, Lord, J. and Ochocka, J. (2001), *Shifting the Paradigm in Community Mental Health: Towards Empowerment and Community*, Toronto: University of Toronto Press.

Nylund, M. (2000), *Varieties of Mutual Support and Voluntary Action: A study of Finnish Self-Help Groups and Volunteers*, Helsinki: The Finnish Federation for Social Welfare and Health.

Ramon, S. (1996), *Mental Health in Europe: Ends, Beginnings and Rediscoveries*, London: MIND.

Rappaport, J. (1993), 'Narrative studies, personal stories and identity transformation in the mutual help context', *Journal of Applied Behavioral Science* **29**(2), 239-256.

Rappaport, J. (2000), 'Community narratives: Tales of terror and joy', *American Journal of Community Psychology*, **28**(1), 1-24.

Richardson, A. and Goodman, M. (1983), *Self-Help and Social Care: Mutual Aid Organisations in Practice*. London: Policy Studies Institute.

Riessman, F. (1990), 'Restructuring help: A human services paradigm for the 1990s', *American Journal of Community Psychology*, **18**(2), 221-230.

Romme, M. and Escher, S. (1993), *Accepting Voices*, London: MIND.

Room, R. (1992), 'Healing ourselves and our planet: The emergence and nature of a generalized twelve-step consciousness', *Contemporary Drug Problems*, **19**(Winter) 717-740.

Salzer, M.S., Rappaport, J. and Segre, L. (2001), 'Mental health professionals support of self-help groups', *Journal of Community and Applied Social Psychology*, **11**(1), 1-10.

Smith, A. and Clarke, J. (2003), *Self-harm Self-help/Support Groups: User led Research on Individual's Experience of Attending a Self-harm Self-help/Support Group and the Support Needs of such Groups*, London: Mental Health Foundation.

Suler, J. (1984), 'The role of ideology in self-help groups', *Social Policy*, **14**, 29-36.

Tew. J. (ed.) (In Press) *Social Perspectives of Mental Health*, London: Jessica Kingsley.

Thoburn, J. and Monanco, M. (1987), *Self Help for Parents with Children in Care*, University of East Anglia Social Work Monographs, Norwich: UEA Publications.

Trojan, A. (1989), 'Benefits of Self-Help Groups: A Survey of 232 Members from 65 Disease-Related Groups', *Social Science and Medicine*, **29**(2), 255-232.

Turner-Crowson, J. and Wallcraft, J. (2002), 'The recovery vision for mental health services and research: A British perspective', *Psychiatric Rehabilitation Journal*, **25**(3), 245-254.

Wallcraft, J. and Bryant, M. (2003), *The Mental Health Service User Movement in England*, London: The Sainsbury Centre for Mental Health.

Wann, M. (1995), *Self-Help and Mutual Aid: A Policy for the 21st Century*, London: Institute for Public Policy Research.

White, B.J. and Madara, E.J. (eds) (2002), *The Self-Help Group Sourcebook: Your Guide to Community and Online Support Groups. 7th ed.*, Denville, New Jersey: Saint Clares Health Services.

Wilson, J. (1995), *Two Worlds: Self Help Groups and Professionals*, Birmingham: British Association of Social Workers.

Wright, S. (2004) 'A participatory study with mental health self-help/mutual groups in England', Unpublished funding proposal of the Strategies for Living Team, London: Mental Health Foundation.

Wuthnow, R. (1994), *Sharing the Journey: Support Groups and America's New Quest for Community*, New York: Free Press.

Chapter 11

The Informal Caring Experience: Issues and Dilemmas

Joan Rapaport

Much has been written about carer burden and carers' feelings of exclusion from the professional care team but little attempt has been made to identify a conceptual framework to give meaning to the carer role. This position is paradoxical in view of the centrality of carers in community care and their potential to advocate for appropriate services for the people they care for. This chapter argues that the current carer position needs to be understood in its historical and political contexts and with reference to recent research, introduces a conceptual framework to enhance the positive potential of the carer role.

Carer Position

Most carers are also relatives (CNA, 1997), but friends and neighbours may also provide care. The 2001 population census in England (Office for National Statistics, 2002) records around 6.8 million carers of which approximately 1.5 million are providing care for a relative or friend with mental illness or some form of dementia. Community care statistics reveal that one-quarter of all adults assessed during 2001/02 by mental health services were identified as having an informal carer (ONS/DoH, 2002). Research into schizophrenia (Johnstone *et al.*, 1984; Birchwood and Smith, 1987; Hogman and Pearson, 1995), depression (Kuipers, 1987), manic depression (Hill *et al.*, 1998) and dementia (Levin *et al.*, 1983; Gilhooly, 1987; Twigg, 1992) report carer sacrifices in health, family and social life, employment, leisure and finances. The proportion of carers whose health is adversely affected by caring responsibilities increases with the increased number of hours spent on caring (Office for National Statistics, 2002).

Service users who live apart from their families are stressed by accommodation, financial and practical problems (Shepherd *et al.*, 1994) but receive more support from services (Hogman and Pearson, 1995). This further suggests the high burden on families in providing ongoing care where the service user still lives in the family home. In order to provide effective care carers need recognition, information and support (Dowling, 1995; Fruin, 1998; DoH, 2002), particularly emotional support '... the most important need to meet and the one that can be the most daunting for professionals' (Kuipers, 1993: 208). Contrary to

popular myths, Johnstone *et al.* (1984) and Jones (2001) found that carer relatives
rarely want the person cared for to return to hospital and seek hospital admission
only as a last resort. Family education studies (for example, Falloon *et al.*, 1984;
Buchkremer *et al.*, 1987) and rapid crisis response services (Keeble *et al.*, 1995)
reveal that family involvement in treatment programmes improves outcomes for
service users and reduces rates of hospital admission.

Since the 1990s the Government has introduced a series of initiatives to
support generic and mental health carers *viz* carer involvement in the service user's
care planning (DoH, 1995), an annual assessment of a carer's own needs (Carers
Act, 1995; DoH, 1999a), funding for carer support initiatives (DoH, 1999b) and
carer services (Carers and Disabled Children Act, 2000; DoH, 2002a). Yet in spite
of these initiatives and their political importance in sustaining community care
(Parker and Clarke, 2002), research suggests that carers still feel marginalised by
services and only a minority have received a carer's assessment and had their
identified needs met (Rethink, 2003). Research conducted by EUFAMI (the
European Federation of Associations of Families of Mentally Ill People) suggests
that families in Switzerland, Norway, Spain, and Germany as in Britain feel
isolated and under-supported, especially in times of need (Brand, 2001).

Whilst the sharing of information between mental health professionals and
carers is a crucial component of supporting carers, it raises many problems (Arksey
et al., 2002). A Rethink survey (Rethink, 1999) found that mental health
professionals used confidentiality issues as a reason to withhold information from
carers. The vital act of carer and professional communication is an ethical issue
(Szmukler and Bloch, 1997) of everyday importance (Rapaport, 2002) but is rarely
afforded ethical status. This chapter contends that a conceptual framework to
support professional and carer interaction is currently missing.

Recent History: Policy and Practice from the 1950s

The term 'relative' had greater universal relevance during the asylum era in view
of the family's role in negotiating hospital care. The term 'carer' first appeared in
community care discussions in the 1970s and was not enshrined in law until the
NHS and Community Care Act 1990 (Twigg, 1994). It has gradually taken the
place of the relative.

Ideologies, Prejudice and Carer Solidarity

Relatives were not consulted about the policy shift from hospital to community
care (Ramon, 1985) although the closures had huge implications for families who
discovered by hard experience that admissions were increasingly difficult to
procure. Whilst closure programmes provided for the old long stay (for example
Tomlinson, 1992; Ramon, 1992) there was no re-provision for new long stay
patients. For this group families were left to fill the vacuum of care (Jones, 2001).
Beliefs that the asylums caused mental illness and that much would automatically

disappear when they had closed (Barham and Hayward, 1995) may have contributed to the general policy of laissez-faire.

Beliefs about the causes of mental illness are complex. Physiological studies into genetic causes have so far proved inconclusive, although concordance rates for schizophrenia are higher amongst identical twins than their fraternal counterparts (Davis *et al.*, 1995). The 'anti-psychiatrists' described schizophrenia as a meaningful response within dysfunctional families (see Hailey, 1959; Rycroft, 1985; Laing and Esterson, 1990). Concepts of high expressed emotion (HEE) associated with psychoeducation theories, although deriving from biological models, implicate families in patient relapse. Recent literature links childhood traumas with adult mental illness (Miller, 1987; Mullen *et al.*, 1993) and impaired development (White and Woolett, 1992). Although no one has ever said that relatives intentionally induce mental illness the implication that their behaviour is involved is offensive to families. Orford (1987: 281) observes that the anti-psychiatry theories 'fostered an atmosphere of suspicion and mistrust between families and mental health services'. Whilst studies suggest that mental illness is caused by multiple social and physiological causes (Vaughan and Leff, 1976; Chua and McKenna, 1995; Wickham and Murray, 1997) the negative implications of the anti-psychiatry theories have lingered.

Iodice and Wodarski (1987) attribute the failure of mental health professionals to support individuals and their families to the establishment of carer self-help groups such as Rethink (then the National Schizophrenia Fellowship) in 1976. This development provided the start of political solidarity for families in mental health.

An Empowered Carer?

The nearest relative defined under Section 26 of the Mental Health Act 1983 is identified by a legally determined hierarchy based on British genealogical traditions underpinned by principles of 'kindred and affinity' (NKH, 1959). The 1983 Mental Health Act gave priority to a relative identified in the hierarchy who cares for the patient with the effect that the nearest relative is often also the patient's main carer. The identified relative has discretionary powers to argue for or against hospital admission for the person cared for and in addition where also the carer, rights to carer entitlements (see Box 11.1).

The 1983 Act introduced the mental health-trained Approved Social Worker (ASW), authorised to make decisions about compulsory admission and involve the nearest relative in the statutory process. In exercising their duties ASWs are required to 'gain the confidence of colleagues in the health services with whom they are required to collaborate' (LAC 86(15) para.14). The powers of the nearest relative and ASW interact and in respect of the applicant functions overlap. Policy development has, however, consistently promoted the professional ASW as the preferred applicant to guard against vested interests and protect the nearest relative's relationship with the patient.

Box 11.1

The powers of the Nearest Relative (civil sections of the Mental Health Act 1983)

- To require the local social services authority to direct an ASW to carry out an assessment of a patient to decide whether or not he or she needs compulsory admission (section 13(4))

- To make an application to detain the patient in hospital (section 11(1)) for assessment (section 2) or treatment (section 3)

- To make an application for the patient's reception by the local authority into guardianship (section 11(1); section 7)

- To notify the ASW that he or she objects to an application for admission for treatment or reception into guardianship (section 11(4))

- To seek to discharge the patient from 1) an assessment or treatment order or 2) from guardianship by a written application in the first instance to the hospital managers and in the second, to the local social services authority (section 23).

Where the nearest relative provides regular and substantial care s/he has:

- A right to an assessment of their caring physical and emotional needs, repeated at least on an annual basis (DoH, 1999a).

ASW duties at the point of an assessment under section 13(4) and duties to inform and consult the nearest relative regarding an admission (sections 11(3) and 11(4)) potentially enhance the civil liberties and public protection functions of the nearest relative's powers. Examination of Parliamentary debates reveals that section 13(4) in particular was introduced to secure an early social assessment of the patient's circumstances with a view to seeking the least restrictive alternative to hospital admission (HL 426 556). The nearest relative's powers to object to a treatment section and seek discharge strengthen the role's position to argue for the least restrictive alternative. The nearest relative is identified as a patient safeguard (DHSS, 1976; DHSS, 1981) and is in essence a type of beneficent advocate, although it has not developed on these lines. However, in spite of the critical importance of reciprocation between the ASW and nearest relative to achieve the best outcome for the patient, the Act does not require the local social services authority to publicise information about the two roles.

Problems in Practice

Since its inception under the 1959 Mental Health Act the nearest relative has been marred by the potential for vested interests inherent in close relationships (HC 598

736). Significantly, service user views on the role's merits are divided according to experiences of good (Bradshaw, 1998; Hart, 1998) and difficult (Lindow, 1998) family relationships. The role has been seriously discredited because of the lottery attached to the identification process and weaknesses in the law to remove inappropriate relatives. Under Section 29 of the Mental Health Act 1983 an ASW or another relative identified under Section 26 can apply to the County Court for the nearest relative to be displaced either by the appointment of the appropriate Director of Social Services, or another individual approved by the Court as suitable to act. However, the criteria to displace the nearest relative are based solely on abilities to carry out the functions of the Act and fail to address real-life problems of abusive or disaffected family relationships.

In spite of concerns about allegations of abuse made by the patient against the relative (Hegarty 1989; MHAC, 1991; Rapaport, 1999) essential recommendations made by the Mental Health Act Commission in 1991 to address the deficiencies of the displacement criteria under the Act (MHAC, 1991) were ignored, thus allowing this serious situation to continue. Local authorities have also faced costly and time consuming litigation where relatives have objected to detention or guardianship although the patient has been deemed to be in serious need of treatment (for example R v Wilson and another *ex parte* Williamson [1996] COD 42). In a few instances relatives have challenged the validity of detention because of ASW failures to identify the right relative (for example S-C [1996] 2 WLR 146. These problems have tarnished the nearest relative's image and by association also that of the carer. The case for nearest relative change was finally won with the advent of the Human Rights Act 1998 and litigation that highlighted the role's potential to breach the right to respect for private and family life under Article 8 of the European Convention on Human Rights (ECHR) (JT v UK 26494/95; FC v UK 37344/97). The Government is now committed to reviewing the Act to allow patients to change the nearest relative in reasonable circumstances.

With regard to the positive safeguard potential of the role the picture is equally disappointing. A small body of literature suggests that relatives generally do not know their rights (Hart, 1998; Gregor, 1999; Rapaport, 2002). Research conducted a few years after the Act's introduction involving 42 local authorities (Barnes *et al.*, 1990) found that social services were reluctant to publicise the nearest relative's power to request an assessment (section 13(4)); reservations about nearest relatives abusing their powers were insinuated. Unsurprisingly, the powers are little used (Hogman and Pearson, 1995; Hart, 1998; Gregor, 1999), although applications to discharge may be less rare than assumed (Rapaport, 2000; Shaw, 2003). The outcomes of research into assessments under the Act (Barnes *et al.*, 1990; Keeble *et al.*, 2000; Quirk *et al.*, 2000; SSI, 2001) support the case that ASWs more generally practise risk avoidance, whilst risk-taking models that exploit crisis situations to help service users and their carers to develop their coping strengths, are largely ignored (Ramon, 2002). Yet the successful outcomes of models supporting hospital diversion (Keeble *et al.*, 1995) family group conferencing (Essex County Council, 2002) and a substantial body of psychoeducation literature (for example Falloon *et al.*, 1984; Buchkremer *et al.*,

1987) suggest that more could be done to develop hospital diversion and supportive frameworks that involve relatives and carers. This conclusion is in part further supported by carer preferences for hospital avoidance (Johnstone *et al.*, 1984; Jones, 2001) and a recent six-year study that found discharges by the nearest relative against psychiatric advice were not associated with a poor clinical outcome (Shaw *et al.*, 2003).

Since the 1990s the nearest relative and ASW have operated in a climate of pre-occupations with risk following a spate of highly publicised homicides committed by people with psychiatric histories. Most of the victims were relatives or associates of the perpetrator (Reith, 1998). These incidents have contributed to increased use of compulsion (Wall *et al.*, 1999), an emphasis on the 'social policing' role of mental health workers, and a culture of blaming professionals when tragedies occur (HC 262 193). Although the numbers of psychiatric homicides are proportionately small and actually declining (Taylor and Gunn, 1999) they continue to have a powerful impact on the media, policy and professional practice. The introduction of powers to supervise patients in the community (section 25A-J) and expansion in medium secure provision are key public protection strategies. Whilst Section 25A-J identifies the carer as the prime consultee over the nearest relative, it also gives the applicant role to the psychiatrist which demonstrates the Government's preference for medical authority over lay and social worker roles. Problems of community re-provision (Ramon, 2000) were not a prime concern.

In addition, during the last decade most ASWs moved from working in local authority teams to multi-agency Community Mental Health Teams (CMHTs). The ASW's professional independence from the psychiatrist is no longer apparent to carers and service users (Hogman and Pearson, 1995; Barnes *et al.*, 2000). Shortages in ASW numbers are reported (MHAC, 1999) and whilst community services have diversified and increased, real alternatives to hospital are still lacking (Barnes *et al.*, 2000). The fact that the ASW is invariably unable to offer a different service also reinforces the role's appearance of conformity with the healthcare team. The ASW's 'wider' responsibilities to support individuals and their families in crisis, and seek alternatives to hospital (LAC 86(15)) have been clipped by political factors and service reconfiguration as well as resource and personnel shortages. These developments have inevitably affected the effectiveness of both nearest relative and carer roles.

Theoretical Frameworks and Legislative Reform

The Government appointed an Expert Committee to advise on legislative reform (DoH, 1999c). The White Paper (DoH, 2000) and subsequent draft Bill (DoH, 2002b) aroused hostile criticism for widening the grounds for compulsion and weakening patient safeguards (MHA, 2003; Church of England, 2003). However, legislative reform was been delayed to allow for a further period of consultation between the Government and stakeholders.

The second Mental Health Bill (Cm 63051-1) and its accompanying Explanatory Notes (Cm 6305-11) was issued on 8th September 2004. This Bill confirms the recommendations of the Expert Committee to replace the nearest relative and ASW roles under a future Act. Under the proposals the nearest relative will be replaced by the roles of nominated person and carer. The latter will be appointed by the patient subject to the approval of the approved mental health professional (AMHP) who replaces the ASW. The carer and nominated person (who may be one and the same) will have rights that even when combined in no way equate with the nearest relative's powers. The new roles overlap but are distinguished in that the carer has the right to request an assessment of the patient whereas the nominated person can appeal to a new tribunal, convened within 28 days of admission, on the patient's behalf. Both roles have rights to be consulted about care plans and discharge, and staff will have duties to provide information about services and how these can be accessed. However, of great significance to carers, professional discretion to exclude the carer from consultations is also proposed especially where to do so would be:

> inappropriate or counter-productive, e.g. where there is conflict of interest or disagreement between the patient and her or his carer (Cm 6305-11: para 55).

'Paragraph 55' considerably reduces the new carer's position in comparison with the statutory authority of the nearest relative and also possible opportunities for helping the patient and his or her carers to address important issues through crises. It also threatens the continuance of traditional social work responsibilities towards individuals and their families currently located in the ASW (LAC 86(15)) and nearest relative roles. The prevalence of an underlying hard attitude towards mental health carers is also suggested that conflicts sharply with the carer policies, already identified, expressly introduced to raise the carer profile.

Principles and Purpose

The Government rejected the Expert Committee's recommendations to incorporate principles including reciprocity into the proposed legislation, although it now seems that these will probably feature in a code of practice to the Act. The Committee's wish to include reciprocity in future legislation was to compensate compulsory patients with appropriate services. However, reciprocity has wider relevance in terms of social interaction and role recognition that are embedded in the nearest relative functions under the current Act.

The proposals confirm the downward trend of the nearest relative, rise of the carer and in respect of the nominated person recognition of patient autonomy, in keeping with contemporary healthcare policy. The replacement of the ASW with the AMHP, a qualified mental health professional such as a social worker or nurse, confirms the loss of the ASW's prerogative, and the ascendance of the multi-disciplinary working.

The nearest relative evolved without an overarching theoretical framework or set of governing principles to shape its development. Although the proposals to remove the nearest relative were made in the absence of research evidence, its likely demise suggests it has not been seen as a resounding success. The role of the carer also lacks a clear theoretical position and under proposed legislation is in addition potentially competing with the nominated person. Furthermore, interpretations of overprotection associated with care arguably conflict with the ideals of patient independence (Twigg, 1994) and patient autonomy. Yet many service users rely on their families for practical and emotional support and want their families to be educated about mental illness and its implications (Shepherd *et al.*, 1994) and helped (Rapaport, 2002). The unclear theoretical position of the nearest relative and carer contrasts sharply with independent advocacy, which the Government has been persuaded to incorporate for patients detained under the new Act.

Advocacy was underpinned by the allied principles of normalisation (Nirje, 1969; Wolfensberger, 1972) and social role valorisation (SRV) (Wolfensberger, 1983) that promoted the need for disadvantaged groups to be enabled to lead lives valued by themselves and the society in which they live. SRV essentially promotes role enhancement and is extensively associated with de-institutionalisation of people with mental health problems. However, Ramon (1991) observes that reciprocity is an essential element of the theory. In short, SRV can only be meaningful if relationships are seen as mutually rewarding and reciprocal. Whilst SRV has neglected carers (Brown and Smith, 1992) and has not been directly related to the nearest relative, reciprocation inherent within the powers provides potential for role valorisation. The debates preceding the role's introduction suggest that it was then considered as a type of beneficent advocacy (HC 562 1696–97). The ethereal influence of SRV on the reciprocal functions of the nearest relative and ASW is arguably also apparent in the 1983 Act changes. However, whereas advocacy has been supported by an explicit theoretical framework and thrived, the nearest relative has been neglected in this regard and is near its demise. This situation has important lessons for the future carer role.

Nearest Relative Research

Recent research into the role of the nearest relative conducted by the author as a PhD (Rapaport, 2002) used focus group interviews to investigate the values, attitudes and actions of carers, service users and ASWs regarding the nearest relative and views about the need for change. The research findings, theoretical development and recommendations are described in greater depth in Rapaport (2002, 2004). The following account provides an overview.

Nearest Relative Problems

The research findings confirmed the problems associated with the identification process including disaffected relationships, the potential for vested interests, and the weaknesses of the system to remove inappropriate relatives. Critically, ASWs reported problems identifying carer relatives especially where the patient was living independently or relationships were estranged, in some cases because of the effects of mental illness. The process could also impose an unwanted burden particularly on carer relatives who had lost their partners. Most significantly, relatives did not use their powers because they did not know about the role. Where they had approached CMHTs for crisis help they had been turned away because nursing staff were also ignorant about the role, in particular Section 13(4). These ostensibly champion carers felt that if they had known about this power very actual and near tragedies might have been avoided. The research also revealed carer and service user difficulties in recalling nearest relative information although it was explained in a variety of formats.

Nearest Relative Potential

Whilst negative stories dominated those highlighting the role's intended positive potential also emerged. A few examples of nearest relatives using their powers to object to a treatment section revealed how the role can dramatically influence the power balances within the team by combining with the ASW to counterbalance medical power. The application of nearest relative and ASW reciprocation caused an effective halt on an otherwise automatic admission and a hard re-assessment of the situation. In one such case an ASW had also clearly gained the support of his own care team to divert the patient from hospital.

The story of the ASW in question is significant because it provides a classic example of the aspirations surrounding the social work contribution under the 1983 Mental Health Act. The patient was already in hospital under section 2. The consultant psychiatrist wanted her to be detained under section 3 for treatment. However, the husband objected and explained that his wife's distress was caused by the death of her baby some ten years previously. The psychiatrist wanted the husband displaced as nearest relative so that the section 3 application could proceed. However, the ASW pointed out that the husband's stance could not be seen as unreasonable and therefore an application to displace him as nearest relative was not only inappropriate, but would also be unlikely to succeed. The ASW focused all his efforts on negotiating a highly intensive network of community care so that the patient could be treated and supported at home.

Kenneth [ASW] '... it depends on their circumstances because you deal with a lot of emotion there and then. I mean funnily enough I had one recently where a nearest relative objected and so I supported him against the doctors and luckily with a lot of consultation we managed to work through an alternative plan of action which was quite involved in terms of this person who proved to, because she was in hospital, she was on a section 2, it was going to be made up to section 3, and we managed to get a care package together with a consultant in the area, reviewed it after a week and did another domiciliary visit and it worked. It did work.'

Senior ASW 'I think what's very interesting about that one is that Kenneth did a massive amount of work in actually what was an alternative to hospital. I know she started off in hospital but it became an alternative to hospital. ... Because she didn't remain on section as intended. And in a way that was because the husband, the nearest relative was objecting ...' (Rapaport, 2002: 271).

In the above case scenario nearest relative status and recognition empowered the husband to explain the tragedy surrounding his wife's distress. The ASW, also empowered by the husband's stance, validated the psychosocial circumstances surrounding the patient's history and galvanised the care team to stretch resources 'to the hilt' to provide alternatives to hospital (Rapaport, 2002: 270). In such cases, in spite of the current risk-conscious climate and scarce resources, the ASW was enabled to apply with rigour the principle of least restriction and seek community solutions.

However, ASW and nearest relative reciprocation had further useful applications. An ASW was able to arrange a full consultation with a consultant psychiatrist for a nearest relative who had objected to a treatment section. The patient had almost died because of a rare reaction to medication and her mother was distraught about the prospects of further treatment. As a result of the consultation the mother was reassured and allowed the section to be instated. In another example, echoing Kuiper's observations about the huge emotional needs of carers and families (*ibid.*, 1993), an ASW trainee recounted the benefits of visiting carer nearest relatives after an admission to allow them to air their distress. The carers felt appreciated: their appreciation reflected on the ASW's feelings that she was fulfilling a much-needed role. Unfortunately, once a fully-fledged ASW, she was unable to provide the same level of commitment because of pressures on her time.

Maria ASW 'I haven't had a lot of problems with the nearest relative but the thing I would like to do is give them more time sometimes. Because I've actually, the sections that I've done have been first time sections and they're quite young people. And sometimes it's the first time the nearest relative has gone through having had contact with mental health services. And sometimes I think they need more time to talk over what's happening to them ... but what came in very useful when I was on ASW training, that we could go back and speak to the relative, but, that actually met quite a few people's needs. But now I'm back at work, I really don't have time to go back and actually speak to people about, you know, about what's going on for them really. Even though I've left my number and said you can, you can call me, but oh, they do call but not to spend hours to speak to, because, you know, you just don't have time really. ... Some kind of tender loving care for them as well ...' (Rapaport, 2002: 280).

Finally, one scenario demonstrated the huge potential of the carer's assessment to highlight not only the carer's needs, but also to give all the professionals involved extra insight into the patient's problems. The patient in question had quite recently been discharged from hospital on his appeal against detention to the hospital managers.[1] However, his mental health deteriorated within days and his parents (who unusually were clearly very aware of their rights) asked

---

[1] The detaining authority has powers to discharge a patient under section 23 of the Mental Health Act 1983.

for an assessment under section 13(4) with a view to his readmission under section. The patient again appealed against his detention to the hospital managers. His parents were clearly concerned that their son would once again be prematurely discharged to their care and asked for a carer's assessment in preparation for the tribunal hearing. This enabled them to explain their side of the story and provide the care team with clearer information about the patient's behaviour.

Larry [ASW] 'There's one case recently where I had to address it [carer's assessment] for a mental health appeal, a manager's appeal and it concentrated very, it concentrated on it a lot because the managers actually discharged the person on one occasion and ten days later the nearest relative requested an assessment. And the person was admitted to hospital and again appealed. So I had to do a fairly extensive report for the managers' meeting. And you know, taking into account the real needs of the carer, to such an extent that when the person actually saw it himself, he withdrew his appeal. When they actually saw that, what was the dynamics that was going on and the needs of the carer ... they sort of came back that they realised themselves, you know, they were getting a little bit more insight ...' (Rapaport, 2002: 280).

As a double bonus, due to the information arising from the carer's assessment and communication between the family, patient and care team, the patient discovered, apparently for the first time, how his behaviour was affecting his parents, with salutary outcomes. He agreed he needed more treatment and withdrew his appeal against detention. The above scenario is particularly interesting because it suggests a process of interaction that bears some resemblance to family education models identified above under 'Carer position'.

Theoretical Development

The research analysis suggests the ethereal influence of SRV with its embedded principle of reciprocity in the nearest relative changes introduced under the 1983 Act. The positive examples of nearest relative and ASW reciprocation for the patient's welfare enhanced the profile of both roles in the eyes of the multi-disciplinary team, the patient and also the ASWs and relatives concerned. The research introduced the term Reciprocal Role Valorisation (RRV) as a new theoretical framework to explain mutual role enhancement (see Box 11.2).

Box 11.2

RRV was found to occur *where the nearest relative and ASW supported each other to achieve mutually respected and identified goals to help the patient, that were recognised by the professionals and significant others involved.* Where the nearest relative and ASW were not working together effectively (or at all) the opposite occurred (Rapaport, 2002: 313).

RRV is conceptually based on the principles of normalisation and SRV. The nearest relative study (Rapaport, 2002) is unique in demonstrating the relevance of SRV theory to not only nearest relatives, but also to carers in mental health and also generic services. This was achieved through the examination of the specific functions of the nearest relative from the perspectives of the three stakeholders most closely involved, *viz* carers, service users and ASWs. RRV provided an overarching framework to support the positive intentions of the nearest relative role and its relationship with the ASW, quintessentially:

- Crisis response
- Least restriction
- Communication and consultation
- Multi-disciplinary working.

However, the research also revealed that negative perceptions of the nearest relative role dominated largely due to the political neglect of the problems surrounding the identification process. These masked the potential of an otherwise valuable role.

Conclusion

Carers in mental health are a vital component of community care who need emotional and practical support to enable them to fulfil their potential. Whilst much has been written about the carer's perspective, the carer role like the nearest relative currently lacks a coherent framework to clarify, shape and maintain its positive objectives. The most pressing challenge for carers in mental health is to ensure that their role is strengthened by a theoretical framework, clear role purpose and also monitoring systems in which they are closely involved. The nearest relative research also revealed the importance of information not only to carers but also professionals and service users about the role, and the centrality of ethics in carer involvement in mental healthcare.

The moral ground of professional and carer ethics urgently needs to be developed to guard against the neglect and overlooked potential of the nearest relative recurring in two new overlapping roles under a future Mental Health Act. RRV is offered as a theoretical starting point as a basis to develop professional and carer reciprocation and mutual recognition and respect.

References

Arksey, H., O'Malley, L. and Harris, J., *et al.* (2002), *Services to Support Carers of People with Mental Health Problems* (NCCSDO), York, University of York.
Barnes, M., Bowl, R. and Fisher, M. (1990), *Sectioned Social Services and the 1983 Mental Health Act*, London, Routledge.

Barham, P. and Hayward, R. (1995), *Relocating Madness, from the Mental Patient to the Person*, London, Free Association Books.

Birchwood, M. and Smith, J. (1987), Schizophrenia and the Family, in: Orford, J. (ed.), *Coping with Disorder in the Family*, London, Croom Helm, 7-38.

Bradshaw, F. (1998), 'I was screaming, I shouldn't be here', *Big Issue*, 5-11, January, 20.

Brand, U. (2001), 'European Perspectives: A carer's view', Acta *Psychiatrica Scandinavica*, 410, 1-6.

Brown, H. and Smith, H. (1992), 'Assertion, not assimilation: A feminist perspective on the normalisation principle', in Brown, H. and Smith, H. (eds), *Normalisation: A reader for the nineties*, London, Routledge, 149-171.

Buchkremer, G., Kinberg, S., Holk, R., Schulze Monking, H. and Hornung, W. (1987), 'Psychoeducational psychotherapy for patients and their key relatives or care-givers: Results of a 2-year follow-up', *Acta Psychiatrica Scandinavia*, Vol. 96, 483-498.

Carers (Recognition and Services) Act 1995.

Carers and Disabled Children Act 2000.

Chua, S. and McKenna, P. (1995), 'Schizophrenia – a Brain Disease? A Critical Review of Structural and Functional Abnormality in the Disorder', *British Journal of Psychiatry*, 6, 563-582.

Church of England (2003), *Emerging Issues in Mental Health*, report by the Mission and Public Affairs Division, London, Church of England.

Cm 6305 – 1 Mental Health Bill 2004.

Cm 6305 – 11 Mental Health Bill Explanatory Notes.

DHSS (1976), *Consultative Document, A Review of the Mental Health Act 1959*, London, HMSO.

DHSS (1981), *Reform of the Mental Health Legislation*, London, HMSO.

DoH (1995), *Building Bridges: Guide to the Arrangements for the Inter-Agency Working for the Care and Protection of Severely Mentally Ill People*, London, HMSO.

DoH (1999a), *National Service Frameworks for Mental Health*, London, Department of Health.

DoH (1999b), *Caring about Carers: National Strategy for Carers*, London, Department of Health.

DoH (2000), *Reforming the Mental Health Act Part 1: The new legal framework*, Cm 5016-1, London, Stationery Office.

DoH (2002a), *Developing services for carers and families of people with mental illness*, London, Department of Health.

DoH (2002b), Draft Mental Health Bill, Cm 5538-I, London, Department of Health.

DoH (2002c), Draft Mental Health Bill Explanatory Notes, London, Department of Health.

Dowling, M. (1995), *A Qualitative Study of Mental Health Service Users' and Carers' Experiences of Community Care*, Royal Holloway College, University of London.

Essex Social Services Department (2002), Essex Family group Conference in Mental Health, Essex County Publications.

Falloon, I., Boyd, J. and McGill, C. (1984), *Family Care of Schizophrenia*, New York, Guilford Press.

FC v. United Kingdom (1999), ECHR, Application No. 37344/97.

Fruin, D. (1998), *A Matter of Chance for Carers? Inspection of local authority support for carers. SSI social care group*, London, Department of Health.

Gilhooly, L. (1987), 'Senile Dementia in the Family', in: Orford, J. (ed.), *Coping with Disorder in the Family*, London, Croom Helm, 138-166.

Gregor, C. (1999), *An Overlooked Stakeholder? The Views of the Nearest Relative on the Mental Health Act Assessment*, Anglia Polytechnic University and Suffolk Social Services.

Hailey, J. (1959), 'The family of the schizophrenic: A model system', *Journal of Nervous Disorders*, 29, 357-374.

Hart, L. (1998), 'Nearest and dearest', *Openmind 94*, 14 December.

HC 562 1696–97, Hansard.

HC 262 193, Hansard.

HC 598 737 Hansard.

Hegarty, D. (1989), 'Escape from a nearest relative', *Social Work Today*, Volume 20, No. 3, 20-21.

HL 426 556, Hansard.

Hill, R., Shepherd, G. and Hardy, P. (1998), 'In sickness and in health: The experiences of friends and relatives caring for people with manic depression', *Journal of Mental Health*, 7. 6, 611-620.

Hogman, G. and Pearson, G. (1995), *The Silent Partners The needs and experiences of people who provide informal care to people with a severe mental illness*, Kingston on Thames, National Schizophrenia Fellowship.

Iodice, J. and Wodarski, J. (1987), 'Aftercare Treatment for Schizophrenics Living at Home, Social Work', 32;2; 122-128.

Johnstone, E., Owens, D., Gold, A., Crow, T. and MacMillan, J.F. (1984), 'Schizophrenic Patients Discharged from Hospital – A Follow-up Study', *British Journal of Psychiatry*, 145, 585-590.

Jones, D. (2001), *Myths, Madness and the Family, The impact of mental illness on families*, London, Macmillan.

JT v. United Kingdom (1997), ECHR, Application No. 26494/95 (reported in Legal Action, 16 July).

Keeble, P., Metcale, C., Riley, T., Waterson, J. and Winter, D. (1995), What users and significant others think about Barnet's Mental Health Crisis Intervention Service, A report from the Crisis Intervention Research Group. London Borough of Barnet.

Kuipers, L. (1987), Depression in the Family, in: Orford, J. (ed.), *Coping with Disorder in the Family*, London, Croom Helm, 194-226.

Kuipers, L. (1993), 'Family burden in schizophrenia; implications for services', *Journal of Social Psychiatry and Epidemiology*, 28, 207-210.

LAC 86(15) *Mental Health Act 1983 – Approved Social Workers*, London, Department of Health and Social Security.

Laing, R. and Esterson, A. (1970), *Sanity, Madness and the Family*, London, Penguin Books.

Levin, E., Sinclair, I. and Gorbach, P. (1983), *The Supporters of Confused Elderly People at Home*, London, National Institute of Social Work.

Lindow, V. (1998), Threats and promises. *Openmind 94*, November/December, 11.

Mental Health Act 1959.

Mental Health Act 1983.

MHA (2003), *Mental Health Alliance Response to the Consultation on Proposed Mental Health Act Reforms*, London, Rethink/Mind.

MHAC (1991), *Mental Health Act Commission 4th Biennial Report 1997–1999*, London, HMSO.

MHAC (1999), *Mental Health Act Commission 8th Biennial Report 1989–1991*, London, HMSO.

NHS and Community Care Act 1990.

Miller, A. (1987), *The Drama of Being a Child*, London, Virago Press.

Mullen, P., Martin, J., Anderson, J., Romans, S. and Herbison, G. (1993), 'Childhood Sexual Abuse and Mental Health in Adult Life', *British Journal of Psychiatry*, 163, 721-732.

Nirje, B. (1969), 'The Normalisation Principle and its Human Management implications', in: Kugel, R. and Wolfensberger, W. (eds), *Changing Patterns in Residential Services for The Mentally Retarded*, Washington President's Committee on Mental Retardation, 255-287.

NKH (1959), *Drafts of the Mental Health Act, Volumes 1-12*, London, Office of Parliamentary Counsel.

Office of National Statistics (2002), *Carers 2000 General Household Survey*, London, HMSO.

Office of National Statistics/DoH (2002), *Community Care Statistics 2000/2001, Referrals, Assessments and Packages of Care for Adults: Report of the findings of the first year of the rollout of RAP*, London, Office of National Statistics.

Orford, J. (1986), 'Integration: A General Account of Families Coping with Disorder', in Orford, J. (ed.), *Coping with Disorder in the Family*, London, Croom Helm; 266-293.

Parker, G. and Clarke, C. (2002), 'Making ends meet: Do carers and disabled people have a common agenda?', *Policy and Politics*, Vol. 30, no. 3, 347-359.

Quirk, A., Lelliott, P., Audini, B. and Buston, K. (2000), What really goes on in Mental Health Act assessments? Findings from an observational study, in Shaping the new Mental Health Act: Key messages from the Department of Health research programme. Royal College of Psychiatrists Study Day, 6 March 2000, 19-21.

Ramon, S. (1985), *Psychiatry in Britain: Meaning and Policy*, London, Gower.

Ramon, S. (1991), 'Principles and Conceptual Knowledge', in: Ramon, S. (ed.), *Beyond Community Care Normalisation and Integration Work*, Basingstoke, Macmillan Press Ltd, 6-33.

Ramon, S. (1992), 'Being at the receiving end of the closure process. The worker's perspective: Living with ambiguity, ambivalence and challenge', in: Ramon, S. (ed.), *Psychiatric Hospital Closure, Myths and Realities*, London, Chapman Hall, 83-121.

Ramon, S. (2000), *A Stakeholder's Approach to Innovation in Mental Health Services A reader for the 21st Century*, Brighton, Pavillion.

Ramon, S. (2002), From Risk Avoidance to Risk Taking Mental Health Social Work, paper presented at the BASW Mental Health conference, *Modernising Mental Health – Shaping the Future*, 20 November, Cambridge, Anglia Polytechnic University.

Rapaport, J. (2000), 'Survey of the Institute of Mental Health Act Practitioners – The use of the Nearest Relative Powers, Detention and Discharge', *The Care Programme Association*, Issue 15, 11-13 October.

Rapaport, J. (2002), A Relative Affair: The Nearest Relative under the Mental Health Act 1983, PhD thesis, Cambridge, Anglia Polytechnic University.

Rapaport, J. (2004), On principle: The Nearest Relative Under the Mental Health Act 1983, www.spn.org.uk.

Reith, M. (1998), *Community Care Tragedies: A Practice Guide to Mental Health Inquiries*, Birmingham, Venture Press.

Rethink (1999). *Information Provision to MH Service Users and Informal Carers*, London, Rethink severe mental illness.

Rethink (2003), *Under Pressure, The Impact of Caring on People Supporting Family Members or Friends with Mental Health Problems*, London, Rethink.

R v. Wilson and another *ex parte* Williamson [1996] COD 42.

Rycroft, C. (1985), *A Critical Dictionary of Psychoanalysis*, London, Penguin Books. S-C [1996] 2 WLR 146.

Shaw, P., Hotopf, M. and Davies, A. (2003), 'In relative danger? The outcome of patients discharged by their nearest relative from sections 2 and 3 of the Mental Health Act', *Psychiatric Bulletin*, Vol. 27, 50-54.

Shepherd, G., Murray, A. and Muijen, M. (1994), *Relative Values, The Differing Views of Users, Family Carers and Professionals on Services for People with Schizophrenia in the Community*, London, Sainsbury Centre.

SSI (2001), *Detained: SSI Inspection of Compulsory Mental Health Admissions*, London, Department of Health.

Szmukler, G. and Bloch, S. (1997), 'Family involvement in the care of people with psychoses: An ethical argument', *British Journal of Psychiatry*, 171, 401-405.

Taylor, P. and Gunn, M. (1999), 'Homicides by People with Mental Illness: Myth and reality', *British Journal of Psychiatry*, 174, 9-14.

Tomlinson, D. (1992), 'Planning after a closure decision: The case for North East Thames Regional Health Authority', in, Ramon, S. (ed.), *Psychiatric Hospital Closure. Myths and Realities*, London, Chapman Hall, 49-82.

Twigg, J. (1992), *Carers Research and Practice*, London, HMSO.

Twigg, J. (1994), 'Carers, Families and Relatives: Socio-legal Conceptions of Care-giving Relationships', *Journal of Social Welfare and Family Law*, Vol. 3, 279-98.

Vaughan, C. and Leff, J. (1976), 'The Influence of Family Social Factors on the Course of Psychiatric Illness', *British Journal of Psychiatry*, 129; 125-137.

Wall, S., Hotopf, M., Wessley, S. and Churchill, R. (1999), 'Trends in the use of the Mental Health Act: England: 1984–96', *British Medical Journal*, Vol. 318, 1520-1521.

White, D. and Woolett, A. (1992), *Families: A Context for Development*, London, Falmer Press.

Wickham, H. and Murray, R. (1997), 'Can biological markers identify endophoenotypes predisposing to schizophrenia?', *International Review of Psychiatry*, 9, 355-364.

Wolfensberger, W. (1972), *The Principle of Normalisation in Human Services*, Toronto, National Institute in Mental Retardation.

Wolfensberger, W. (1983), Social Role Valorisation: A Proposed New Term for the Principle of Normalisation, Vol. 21, no. 6, 234-239.

Chapter 12

Living with Trauma

Janet E. Williams

Introduction

Since the Ancient Greeks there has been a common sense understanding that extreme situations and events can lead to extreme human responses: those noted were mostly in the public domain such as war or large scale catastrophes. In the last few decades this has become accepted within the field of mental health, with theories of explanation coming predominantly from psychiatry and psychology based upon either symptom orientation or construct approaches. Latterly, aspects of more commonly lived experience have been identified as potentially traumatic by reason of their oppressive nature, such as racism and violence in the home towards women and children. This chapter considers how all these perspectives contribute, in a contested field, to informing the development of a psychosocial approach to working with survivors of trauma, with particular reference to women survivors of child sexual abuse (CSA) and refugees.

The recognition of trauma as a concept was delayed for several reasons. There was controversy about where responsibility should lie, externally or within the individual, since this was relevant for compensation claims (van der Kolk, McFarlane *et al.*, 1996: x). The significant reason lies in the dominance of the medical profession which would not legitimate it until it had been *produced* as a diagnosis within the bio-medical paradigm. This occurred after the Vietnam War, when Post Traumatic Stress Disorder (PTSD) was added to the Diagnostic and Statistical manual of Mental Disorders (DSM) in 1980 by the American Psychiatric Association and further refined in 1987 (DSM-III-R). It appears also in the ICD-10 diagnostic category (International Classification of Diseases). Since then the diagnosis has been widely used, researched and it limits identified such that is now sometimes referred to as Type 1 or simple trauma. Within the bio-medical paradigm a Type 11 or more complex form has been proposed for enduring traumatic situations such as child sexual abuse or victimisation from war crimes (Terr, 1991; Joseph, Williams *et al.*, 1997). Though widely used it is not formally recognised within psychiatry (Amaya-Jackson, Davidson *et al.*, 1999; Goodman, Thompson *et al.*, 1999; Williams, 2002).

Understanding Trauma

The Medical Model of Trauma – PTSD

PTSD, as a medical category remains a narrowly defined concept, or disorder, with a specific list of symptoms. Medical hegemony in mental health has thus restricted the parameters for trauma research and practice in order to comply with this positivist/scientific paradigm; this has been criticised as a medicalisation of what are often social problems (Kelly, 1989; Smail, 1993: 12).

This diagnosis relies upon a single event, such as a natural disaster, physical assault, sudden death, or witnessing of death or violence, with a precise duration of response. The individual must have experienced or witnessed this sort of event with a response of intense fear, helplessness or horror, resulting in intense anxiety, confusion and depression. Not included are well recognised traumatic events such as threats to the individual's psychic integrity or sense of self, or of severe, uncontrollable psychological pain (Carlson and Dalenburger, 2000).

The other criteria are:

- intrusive and recurrent reliving of the event and intense psychological distress to cues that symbolise or resemble it
- persistent avoidance of stimuli associated with the trauma or numbing of general responsiveness including, lack of recall of important aspects of the trauma feelings of detachment and the sense of a foreshortened future
- persistent symptoms of increased arousal including, difficulties sleeping
- irritability or outbursts of anger, difficulty concentrating, hyper-vigilance or exaggerated startle response.

As with all diagnoses a checklist may provide a useful aide-memoire, or alternatively as method of categorising or validating someone's claims of distress. A number of psychological tests have been designed with this latter purpose, that is to provide a standardised, quantifiable external view of the severity of the trauma, one such is the Impact of Event Scale (IES) (Horowitz *et al.*, 1979) or Saunders *et al.* (1990) 28 item scale for crime related post-traumatic stress. In contrast, many other mental health professionals start with the person's own narrative and expressions of distress in order to determine whether that person, in their own terms, has been traumatised.

Psychological Models of Traumatic Stress

Psychological approaches generally use the PTSD classification, or a modified version, as a starting point. Though a symptom based approach is used, such as the Scales mentioned above, the psychological literature is concerned with meaning given to experiences and thereby explaining the adaptations made to trauma through coping mechanisms. Current theories include:

- the science of memory and dissociation (Hacking, 1994; Herman, 1992; Van der Kolk, McFarlane *et al.*, 1996; Hall, 2000)
- the distortion of the maturation process in childhood (Briere, 2002; Finkelhor and Browne, 1985)
- world views and schema known as construct approaches (Horowitz, 1983; Hall, 2000; Briere, 2002).

Dissociation is understood to be a mechanism used at the time of the trauma, to a lesser or greater degree, in order to protect the individual from being overwhelmed. This enables the person to be elsewhere during the experience through psychologically separating themselves from it, and separating out the elements of the event. This results in the memory of it being fragmented such that no integrated comprehensive account of the events(s) is stored. This means that full recall of events, or meaningful memory that can be verbalised, are inaccessible often for long periods of time. If the trauma was experienced before language was acquired then it may never be fully recalled or put into words. With dissociation may come the intrusion of fragments of memory, usually incomprehensible to the individual and to others because they are incomplete and not associated with any remembered events. Such unwanted recall is confusing and often distressing. Dissociation, in some circumstances, may become an automatic rather than a chosen response.

Though widely used, the focus on dissociation has been criticised as being conceptually ambiguous and when used to the exclusion of other approaches potentially pathologising (Feiring, Taska *et al.*, 1996; Hall, 2000; Wyatt and Newcombe, 1990). The use of the diagnosis 'dissociative identity disorder' (DID), previously described as multiple personality disorder, identifies the person as disorganised, disabled and discredited (Putnam, 1989). This is rooted in a negative evaluation of coping strategies as maladaptive and pathological.

The impact of childhood trauma on adults is often explained by a distortion in the maturation process. Type 11 Trauma has developed as a theory in order to take account of the effect of ongoing, predictable traumatic events in childhood which may prevent the normal, gradual development of social and psychological capacity and distort the development process itself. The psychological literature describes the complex response to trauma for children including the disruption to the development of key skills for dealing with disturbing events and emotions (Briere, 2002). Thus a child, and then the adult, is without the means to deal with difficult emotions and becomes overwhelmed in situations where others may not. Mechanisms such as self harming, particularly cutting and somatisation may be employed as relief in these overwhelming situations. Characteristically these are the behaviours described in the diagnosis of Borderline Personality Disordered (BPD). Less attention may be given to the social consequences, such as poor school performance, which may also leave the individual overwhelmed and powerless in adulthood. This puts survivors of CSA at risk of receiving the diagnosis of Borderline Personality Disorder and approximately 70 per cent of those with this diagnosis are survivors (Meichenbaum, 1994).

A widely used cognitive-behavioural framework is based upon the theory that basic, usually unquestioned assumptions about the world, the person and others – world views or schema – are challenged by the impact of traumatic events (Finkelhor and Browne, 1985; Horowitz, 1983; Parks, 1975). It is thought that most people are likely to have a world view in which they see themselves as fairly invulnerable following a secure and predictable upbringing (Bowlby, 1969; Erikson, 1950). This world view is challenged by an extreme, traumatic event and consequently may be the focus of professional input for those with PTSD (Janoff-Bulman and Frieze, 1983; Perloff, 1983).

It is argued by Janoff-Bulman (1989) that there are two options, the former being easier than the latter:

- Assimilation and integration – changing the construction and understanding of the trauma to make it fit the existing world view
- Accommodation – changing the world view to accommodate the trauma.

The World Assumption Scale (WAS scale) was developed from this to include three categories; benevolence, meaningfulness of the world and worthiness of self. For children it could be argued that both elements, above, may occur and interact, since their world view is still being developed and they are having to construct sense out of the contradictions between events as they experience them and the interpretation of the events from the perpetrator's perspective. For survivors of child sexual abuse (CSA) Hall talks of the world view as core issues such as 'I am nothing' (inconsequential) and 'I am bad/wrong', which she says operate throughout the life stages of women survivors (Hall, 2000). Briere also uses this concept in his Self-trauma Theory to show how significant and embedded the trauma and implicit memories become in the world view, 'basic beliefs that function more as a general model of self and others than as actual thought, per se' (Briere, 2002: 177).

Psychosocial Perspectives on Trauma

There are many outspoken voices which have exposed the shortcomings of taking an approach to trauma and mental health which ignores the significance of societal power, both in producing and maintaining poor mental health (Masson, 1988; Smail, 1993). If the causes are in the outside world they are unlikely to be within the individual's capacity to modify and will remain irrespective of personal change. To equate success with the individual's adaptation to oppressive circumstances will not only set up the person to fail, thus confirming their incapacity, but leave the causes of trauma and distress outside the debate, unchallenged, maintained and hidden. Research and theory in this field come from sources and standpoints such as narrative, critical inquiry, discourse analysis and other social constructionist approaches as well as through emancipatory methodologies where subjects are co-researchers. These predominantly qualitative approaches are particularly well suited to address meanings and perspectives of participants and can offer access to deep structural and interpersonal processes.

The emergence of PTSD represents a safe development as it includes primarily public events. To incorporate the effects of physical and sexual violence towards women and children in the domestic sphere would require stepping outside the scientific paradigm and would embroil bio-medicine in the social complexities of society and family. In most professional education such traumas are not conceptualised in terms of power inequality or masculinity. The corollary is that there exists the same prevalence of racism, sexism and homophobia within mental health services as in the general population (Health, 2002) and similarly no recognition of the prevalence of domestic and sexual violence. Without this knowledge the myths and stereotypes which maintain the culture of the family are unlikely to be challenged, reinforced as they are by the media and bound up in tradition through State and church. The sanctity of family life and personal relationships are maintained by social silence and a professional disquiet about interfering in the private power structures of the family.

Amongst the social movements within mental health there is a recognition that some people want talking therapies, social action to counteract stigma and interventions which have a direct impact upon the quality of life and life chances (Health, 2002). This is the combination which could accurately be described as psychosocial. The aim of the approach is the empowerment of individuals and groups, through attention to the person as a subjective individual through appropriate therapeutic interventions, attention to their social identity, often through collective approaches such as group work, and opportunities for citizenship through influencing service provision and social stigma.

Living with Trauma from Child Sexual Abuse (CSA)

Pat is a working class woman in early 40s living in an ex-pit village. She has three children who no longer live with her. She has a history of unhappy relationships, periodically she drinks heavily and harms herself. Her first contact with mental health services followed the birth of her first child at the age of 18 and she was subsequently admitted compulsorily to a psychiatric hospital. She had other periods of hospitalisation and frequently attended Accident and Emergency services after harming herself by cutting. She continues to be supported in her home by the Community Mental Health Team, attends a day centre, was diagnosed as schizophrenic and later Borderline Personality Disordered and is prescribed anti-psychotic medication and anti-depressants.

This is a common scenario and there are many such women supported by mental health services, in special hospitals and prisons, whose history of abuse has never been disclosed or enquired after. Estimates vary according to cohort and definitions used but it appears that 12-51 per cent of women and 7-16 per cent of men having been sexually abused (Hagan, Donnison *et al.*, 1998) and a disproportionately high percentage of these use mental health services compared with the general population, with a conservative estimate of between 30-50 per cent of the women using services having been abused (Hagan, Donnison *et al.*, 1998). Not all women who have been abused will have lasting effects, some are fortunate to have protective networks or other factors which have built up their resilience during childhood and beyond.

By looking beyond the diagnosis, and encouraging Pat to tell her story, the history of abuse is told and begins to explain her continuing difficulties and the re-victimisation in her personal life. Professionals are hesitant to ask about abuse, but the research shows that women want to be questioned about it and to address it (Health, 2002).

- She was sexually abused by her father and later by her brother. She began to drink heavily in her early teens and finally escaped from home by moving in with the father of her first child. This was an abusive relationship, the first of many
- The intimate procedures during pregnancy and birth triggered memories of the sexual abuse, her jealous partner kept her isolated from her friends and she chose to avoid her abusive family. She became very distressed, lived with constant flashbacks which included hearing voices. This resulted in her first compulsory admission to a psychiatric hospital and the diagnosis of psychosis
- The second period of admissions was triggered by the loss of her significant childhood relationship, her grandmother, and the return of her father to the district. Her eldest daughter was now the same age as she had been when the abuse first started. She was beset with memories and terrified that she could not protect her daughter, but did not dare to reveal the reasons
- The experience of hospital admission was retraumatising because of the close contact with men on the mixed wards, the sexual innuendoes and other bantering that was common amongst male staff and patients. The staff found it difficult and unrewarding working with her when she continued to self-harm and she was often treated with disdain. Her self harming and her apparently uncontrollable mood changes and the lack of progress in mediating her behaviour brought her the diagnosis of Borderline Personality Disorder and no treatment other than containment through anti-depressants and anti-psychotic medication.

Pat suffered from 'a matrix of childhood disadvantages from which abuse emerged' (Mullen, 1996: 7). This occurs across all classes and ethnic groups.

Perpetrators of child sexual abuse calculate the effect of their behaviour on the child and carry out a social process of grooming designed to produce acceptance and then compliance by reducing the child's resistance through the destruction of their self-esteem. Over time the messages are assimilated and the child accommodates by changing their world view so successfully that they may eradicate memories or sense of self before the abuse. Finkelhor and Browne's have summarised the effect of CSA in their Framework of Traumagenic Dynamics, in which they found that the power of the perpetrator is to sexualise, to stigmatise and betray (Finkelhor, 1986).

In more detail we can see that the grooming processes are designed to induce in the child:

- Confusion

  The abuser first sets up a positive relationship which changes to become negative and threatening and changes to be inconsistent with the child whilst being consistent with others.

  The child is told that they are powerful – the cause of the abuse – but feels helpless.

  There is pain and sometimes pleasure.

  The experience may be normalised whilst the child feels it to be abnormal.

  The child loses the capacity to trust in their own interpretations of events and in whom to trust, may confuse love and affection with sexual activity, will be unsure about their own and others personal boundaries and how to keep safe.
- Responsibility for what happens, through misrepresentation and making the child take an active part in the sexual activities, producing guilt and shame.
- Isolation, abandonment and despair: loss of contact from peers and others because their worlds are so different, loss of trust in all relationships as result of betrayal. This may be exacerbated by the calculated actions of the abuser who may make themselves the central source of information for the child and those around them.
- The response may be to withdraw, to be overly clingy and to use sexualised behaviour to gain affection. The child fails to gain family and social skills necessary for negotiating transitions to and during adulthood.
- Internalisation of the shame means that the child is induced to feel bad, dirty, self-hatred and different from the stereotypical family; a process fuelled by popular negative stereotypes of femininity and masculinity.   ·
- Powerless so that it becomes difficult to disclose and change what is happening for fear of violence, implied or real, and psychological pain maintained through enforced silence. Equally the child may be told that the power to seduce is theirs alone whilst the reality is of helplessness. Low self-esteem and poor concentration results in poor performance in school and doubts about capacity to learn (Warner, 2000).

The strategies used by survivors to deal with the effects of this type of trauma are well documented and are seen most often in the expression and containment of pain, shame and distress through substance misuse, depression, self-harm, eating disorders, increased hospitalisation and dissociative problems. Relationally there may be difficulties with trust, intimacy and sexuality often resulting in engagement with retraumatising relationships. Parenting may be more difficult with an increased risk of losing children into the care system (Browne and Finkelhor, 1986; Hurley, 1991; Wyatt, Guthrie *et al.*, 1992; Rorty, Yager *et al.*, 1994; Feiring, Taska *et al.*, 1996; van der Kolk, McFarlane *et al.*, 1996). Survivors are known to be at higher risk for health problems and may be marginalised by characteristics of gender, race, and isolation stemming from the privatised nature of their trauma (Hall, Stevens *et al.*, 1994), their lack of social education and poverty.

Power

A power mapping of Pat's life as both child and adult show little change in many respects; she remains powerless (Hagan and Smail, 1997). This is due to several factors, her social exclusion – she is semi-literate, poor, unemployed and lives in an impoverished social environment – and her psychological difficulties. She deals with her distress through numbing herself with alcohol and prescribed medication, and relieves her emotional numbness by cutting herself. Her body is not under her control when she is in abusive relationships but she has some strategies for dealing with her distress.

The aim of support to Pat is to assist her to move from victim to survivor role, and this requires attention to her powerlessness in the three main spheres of her life: personally and psychologically as a woman within society; within her social networks and at a societal level in terms of access to resources Dalrymple and Burke, 1995; Thompson, 2001; Holland, 1992). She needs what Rapport describes as 'both a psychological sense of personal control or influence and a concern with actual social influence, political power and legal rights' (Rappaport, 1987: 121).

At the level of individual meaning Pat needs access to people who want to hear and understand her as she constructs and questions her life story and forms her own biography in relation to trauma, gender and her social and family experiences. Being believed, lifting the silence and finding a voice is one of the first steps to her empowerment. It also opens up the opportunity to understand the methods she has used to survive her experiences and for her to determine whether these should change. Interventions that do not actively take account of her powerlessness run the danger of retraumatising Pat and at best will not enable her to move on; at worst will add to her sense of failure. For example telling her story does not imply focussing on the traumatic events; rather the interpretation and the beliefs about herself and others which have developed from them; past issues are embedded in current difficulties or strengths where they can be explored. Constructing her story is not about fundamental truths or uncovering a precise story. To compel her to disclose finer and more intimate details and to put these under surveillance will produce more subordination and what Rose describes as the 'colonisation of experiences and understanding ...' (Rose, 1990: 241). This also rules out conventional methods of desensitisation which are commonly used with PTSD. Working with survivors who have not had clear boundaries and who have had the role of victim reinforced for them from childhood, and often through adulthood, requires a clear and explicit focus, whether from support workers, therapists or in group work.

Within the cultural sphere, Pat as a woman can learn about societal assumptions about gender, race, heterosexuality and mental health. This may enable her to question her own socialisation and to aspire for better things as she understands her situation to be in common with many other women. One way to do this is to experience the commonality and solidarity with other women and survivors and to understand the prevalence and mechanisms of abuse as part of a wider social phenomenon in which masculinity is used to justify the submission of children and women through sexual violence. Framing abuse in this social context may reduce the sense of shame, guilt, and feelings of personal failure. Sharing and understanding this in a group breaks the contained silence, counteracts the isolation of childhood and has the potential to open up networks of support, in which all group members can both offer and receive help, thus overturning the status of victim. Community groups and women's groups, which are not stigmatising and are organised around other aspects of her identity, are likely to be useful.

As Pat becomes more at ease with her past she may be able to identify networks of support within her existing social and family circle. Most survivors have periods of needing intense support and the wider the circle the better. To use networks that she owns, either from the past or through community or mutual support groups, validates her own judgements and is a practical demonstration of her capacity to be a survivor rather than a victim.

At societal level Pat needs support to obtain new skills for managing her life, such as literacy and parenting skills as well as knowledge about her rights, education and employment. Most discharged patients, even without the trauma of abuse, have very few resources at their disposal (Hunt and Hemmings, 1991). Improvements in these aspects of her life not only bring material change but represent success which potentially increases self-esteem. Any interventions and support has to take account of a history of powerlessness and her world view which may include a deep insecurity about her capacity to learn. Participation in community networks and adult education services, where others are also learning basic skills, perhaps with the discrete support of mental health professionals, may be appropriate. Intense therapeutic work may not be what she wants and is unlikely to be successful if she is preoccupied by immediate practical problems such as housing, finance or difficulties with her children. Therapy may destabilise her precarious hold on her life.

Living with Trauma from War Crimes

Mohammed is 25, a Kurd who has arrived in the UK. He is one of the 14 million refugees and asylum seekers in the world (Refugees, 2000; Weaver and Burns, 2001). He was tortured and was helped to escape but had to leave the rest of his family in his homeland. He has been traumatised by his experiences, by the difficulties of his migration and this continues as he remains preoccupied with his family's future, and he is received with racism and threats of violence in the South coast town where he has been housed. He has received no help to discuss or deal with the impact of his torture, to integrate into the community and he is forbidden to work. He has, once again, become a member of an identifiable and socially excluded group. In practice, asylum seekers are excluded from access to civic society and ordinary services, sometimes through physical segregation, through the lack of awareness and sensitivity to their specific needs as well as from practical barriers related to lack of information, language difficulties and bureaucracy. Many agencies are still unfamiliar with, or even uninterested in, the needs of asylum seekers whilst others, including health, education and social services are under-prepared and funded to respond adequately.

The trauma experienced by adults such as Mohammed is likely to be different from that suffered by survivors of CSA and PTSD in several respects. Firstly it occurs after the development of his self-identity so he retains his previous, normal world view, unlike survivors of childhood abuse; secondly torture and ongoing or predictable violence is quite different from the single catastrophe that defines PTSD.

Torture is a shock to the individual's world view and assumptions about security, vulnerability and the nature of humankind. The processes used by the State against its citizens, or by invading armies, are as calculated as those of perpetrators of CSA. Torture and related activities are designed to destroy people's sense of self in various ways: through political and social re-education; by instilling a culture of conspiracy through the breakdown of trust within families and communities and through the ever present fear of death or torture for self and kin. Events are taken out of control of the individual and his or her social network. Victims of torture generally have experiences that are so terrible that most people cannot believe them (International, 1997; Weaver, 2001).

For women refugees, the impact of sexual violence as a form of war crime may have stigmatised and excluded them from their family and community networks especially in cultures where a family's virtue is connected to a woman's virginity or monogamy. In the UK, over the last few years, the number of women has increased considerably, as a proportion of those seeking asylum; most of whom have been subject to rape and sexual torture.

Helping to Live with Trauma

Asylum seekers represent one of the poorest and most socially excluded groups in the host society. There is a growing recognition that this is the factor most damaging to their mental health, and that this comprises a significant trauma generated by the uncertainties in the asylum processes and the hostility of the host community. The priority for most asylum seekers is practical help with these issues, the asylum claim, legal assistance, housing, finding their families and accessing health care. Workers in the organisations meeting this need, such as The Refugee Council, community groups, Personal Medical Services are also working with the trauma in practical and often low key ways, through simply listening and sometimes offering counselling.

The approach is often described as public health in which the social factors relating to mental health, and general health, are recognised. For mental health this provides an understanding of the trauma which places it, for most people, within the normal and expected range of responses to terrible events. Thus it is not described as mental illness but rather as psychological difficulties, which the majority of asylum seekers experience. This approach also avoids the additional problems brought about by becoming a user of mental health services and being labelled with a medical diagnosis.

Exclusion from and lack of safety in the communities to which where asylum seekers are dispersed are sources of stress. Community work in some places has been very successful, bringing together young men for example in Hull, through art, cultural events as well as sport. This has brought greater understanding and safety to the incoming community. Community groups, run by refugees and asylum seekers, have the potential to offer advice on accessing services and about the host culture, active and individual support to new arrivals, culturally sensitive listening and advice from peers, campaigning activity to improve services, and skill sharing. Linking refugees into their own communities offers the greatest chance for the ordinary and familiar patterns to be re-established, which Summerfield argues, is the context for recovery, not as a 'discrete process' but as something that

> happens in people's lives rather than in their psychologies. It is practical and unspectacular, and it is grounded in the resumption of the ordinary rhythms of everyday life – the familial, socio-cultural, religious, and economic activities that make the world intelligible (Summerfield, 2002: 1107).

However within this there must be separate safe places for women, since many of them will have experienced sexual violence from men. For others there will be a need for further work, to make sense of the trauma of torture within their world view. This is likely to be related to sexual trauma for women, but there are also many men in this situation. Helping cross culturally with such intensely difficult issues such as torture is a challenge. Firstly counselling, which in the West has become the standard response to personal difficulties, is not accepted in many cultures. The automatic assumption or imposition of this approach is potentially hegemonic and ineffective. In Mozambique, for example, traditional healing mechanisms are used extensively at grass roots level and these do not include talking about traumatic experiences (Hayner, 2001). This is a similar picture for Cambodian refugees in the USA,

> most Cambodians refugees suffer silently. They do not complain about their situations or blame others but for their inability to adjust, and in spite of their difficulties, work hard and try to express an optimistic attitude (Blair, 2001; Strober, 1994: 34).

Both studies show that it was the immediate and extended family that had been the most helpful for adjusting to their new environment, rather than an individualised approach such as counselling.

Torture and related crimes are issues of social and political injustice. Anger and revenge, if viewed as barriers to healing and acceptance, and even to political reconciliation, can invalidate the individual's political aspirations for change and social justice. Counselling has to deal with the past but also the future; the possibility of a failed claim for asylum and how to prepare to return home, as well as the challenge of remaining in the UK if the claim is accepted.

Conclusion

A psychosocial approach to helping people live with trauma takes its lead from the central impact of trauma – powerlessness. Professional relationships with survivors of trauma can only begin through transparent interactions where power and powerlessness are part of both the implicit and explicit processes, where the individual's powerlessness is understood to relate to social inequality not personal failure, and where there is the possibility of developing trust. What helps will vary over time but, whether it be traditional therapeutic interventions or socially based activities, attention is paid to both the structural impact of social exclusion and to individual and collective meaning of the experiences. Psychosocial practice requires the practitioner not only to trust in the expertise of the individual survivor but also to respect, develop and work alongside the person's social networks which are not under the control of mental health services.

Understanding the impact of trauma and responding to it would require a major reorientation of mental health services, away from medically defined categories and priorities which relate to risk rather than levels of distress. With the recognition of the impact of abuse and trauma on survivors comes the recognition of the impact of this work on practitioners, interpreters and family networks. Effective work involves engaging in pain, despair and helplessness and facing unanswerable, existential questions rather than anaesthetising people with medication. Much of this work is already being done, despite the system, by a few committed individuals or small voluntary groups. All those involved need help to avoid being traumatised themselves, to see the issues holistically and to receive recognition, support, supervision, time and training.

References

Amaya-Jackson, L.J., Davidson, R., Hughes, D.C., Swartz, M., Reynolds, V., George, L.K. and Blazer, D.G. (1999), 'Functional impairment and utilization of services associated with posttraumatic stress in the community', *Journal of Traumatic Stress*, 12, 709-724.

Amnesty International (1997), *Refugees: Human Rights have no Borders*, Amnesty International.

Blair, R.G. (2001), 'Mental health needs among Cambodian refugees in Utah', *International Social Work*, 44(2), 179-196.

Bowlby, J. (1969), *Attachment and Loss*, London: Hogarth.

Briere, J. (2002), 'Treating adult survivors of severe childhood abuse and neglect: Further Development on an Integrated Model', in J.E.B. Myers, L. Berliner, J. Briere, C.T. Hendrix, C. Jenny and A.T. Reid (eds), *The American Professional Society on the Abuse of Children Handbook on Child Maltreatment*, London: Sage.

Browne, A. and. Finkelhor, D. (1986), 'The impact of childhood sexual abuse: A review of the research', *Psychological Bulletin*, 99, 66-77.

Carlson, E.B. and Dalenburger, C. (2000). 'A conceptual framework for the impact of traumatic experiences', *Trauma, Violence and Abuse*, 1(1), 4-28.

Dalrymple, J. and Burke, B. (1995), *Anti-Oppressive Practice: Social Care and the Law*, Buckingham: Open University Press.

Erikson, E. (1950), *Childhood and Society*, New York: Norton.

Feiring, C., L. Taska, L. Lewis, M. (1996), 'A process model for understanding adaptation to sexual abuse: The role of shame in defining stigmatization', *Child Abuse and Neglect*, 20, 767-782.

Finkelhor, D. (1986), *A Source Book on Child Sexual Abuse*, London: Sage.

Finkelhor, D. and Browne, A. (1985), 'The traumatic impact of child sexual abuse: A conceptualization', *Journal of Orthopsychiatry*, 55(4), 530-541.

Goodman, L.A., Thompson, K.M., Weinfurt, K., Corl, S., Acker, P., Mueser, K.T. and Rosenberg, S.D. (1999), 'Reliability of reports of violent victimisation and posttraumatic stress disorder among men and women with serious mental illness', *Journal of Traumatic Stress Disorder*, 12, 587-599.

Hacking, I. (1994), *Rewriting the Soul: Multiple Personality and the Sciences of Memory*, Princeton, NJ: Princeton University Press.

Hagan, T., Donnison, J., Gregory, K,. Martindale, S. and Hamnett, M. (1998), *Breaking the Silence: Working with Adult Survivors of Childhood Sexual Abuse*, Brighton: Pavilion Publishing (Brighton) Ltd.

Hagan, T. and Smail, D. (1997), 'Power-Mapping-II. Practical Application: The example of child sexual abuse', *Journal of Community and Applied Social Psychology*, 7, 269-284.

Hall, J.M. (2000), 'Dissociative experiences described by women survivors of childhood abuse', *Journal of Interpersonal Violence* 15(2), 184-204.

Hall, J.M., Stevens, P.E. and Meleis, A.I. (1994), 'Marginalizatioin: A guiding concept for valuing diversity in nursing knowledge development', *Advances in Nursing Science*, 16(4), 23-41.

Hayner, P. (2001), *Unspeakable Truths: Confronting State Terror and Atrocity*, London: Routledge.

Health, D.O. (2002), 'Women's Mental Health: Into the Mainstream: Strategic Development of Mental Health Care for Women', Summary, London: Department of Health.

Herman, J. (1992), *Trauma and Recover*, New York: Basic Books.

Holland, S. (1992), 'From social abuse to social action', in J. Ussher and P. Nicholson (eds), *Gender Issues in Clinical Psychology*, London: Routledge.

Horowitz, M.J. (1983), 'Psychological response to serious life events', in S. Breznitz (ed.), *The Denial of Stress*, New York: International Universities Press.

Hunt, B.J. and Hemmings, A.J. (1991), 'Mentally Ill People in the Community: An Inquiry into the Well-being of the Long-term Mentally Ill in Hastings', University of Sussex: Health Studies Unit, Centre for Medical Research.

Hurley, D.L. (1991), 'Women, alcohol and incest: An analytical review', *Journal of Studies on Alcohol*, 52(3), 253-268.

Janoff-Bulman, R. and Frieze, I.H. (1983), 'A theoretical perspective for understanding reactions to victimization', *Journal of Social Issues*, 39, 1-17.

Joseph, S., Williams, R. and Yule, W. (1997), *Understanding Post-Traumatic Stress: A Psychosocial Perspective on PTSD and Treatment*, Chichester: John Wiley & Sons.

Kelly, L. (1989), 'From politics to pathology: The medicalisation of the impact of rape and child sexual abuse', *Radical Community Medicine: Sexuality*, Winter.

Masson, J. (1988), *Against Therapy*, London: Collins Fontana.

Meichenbaum, D. (1994), *Treating Post-Traumatic Stress Disorder: A Handbook and Practice Manual for Therapy*, Chichester: John Wiley & Sons.

Parks, C.M. (1975), 'What becomes of redundant world models? A contribution to the study of adaptation to change', *British Journal of Medical Psychology*, 48, 131-137.

Perloff, L.S. (1983), 'Perceptions of vulnerability to victimization', *Journal of Social Issues*, 39(2), 41-62.

Putnam, F.W. (1989), *The Diagnosis and Treatment of Multiple Personality Disorder*, New York: Guildford.

Rappaport, J. (1987), 'Terms of empowerment/exemplars of prevention: Toward a theory for community psychology', *American Journal of Community Psychology*, 15(2), 121-44.

US Committee for Refugees (2000), *World Refugee Survey 2000*, Washington DC: Immigration and Refugee Services of America.

Rorty, M., Yager, J. and Rossotto, M.A. (1994), 'Child sexual, physical and psychological abuse in bulimia nervosa', *American Journal of Psychiatry*, 151, 1122-1126.

Rose, N. (1990), *Governing the Soul: The Shaping of the Private Self*, London: Routledge.

Smail, D. (1993), *The Origins of Unhappiness*, London: HarperCollins.

Strober, S. (1994), 'Social Work Interventions to Alleviate Cambodian Refugee Psychological Distress', *International Social Work*, 37, 23-35.

Terr, L.C. (1991), 'Childhood traumas: An outline and overview', *American Journal of Psychiatry*, 148, 10-20.

Thompson, N. (2001), 3rd ed. *Anti-discriminatory Practice*, Palgrave: Basingstoke.

Van der Kolk, B.A., McFarlane, A.C. and Weisaeth, L. (eds) (1996), *Traumatic Stress: The Overwhelming Experience on Mind, Body and Society*, London: The Guildford Press.

Warner, S. (2000), *Understanding Child Sexual Abuse: Making the Tactics Visible*, Gloucester: Handsell Publishing.

Weaver, H.N. and Burns B.J. (2001), '"I shout with fear at night". Understanding the traumatic experiences of refugees and asylum seekers', *Journal of Social Work*, 1(2), 147-164.

Williams, J.E. (2002), *Services Meeting Needs of Female Survivors of Child Sexual Abuse*, Sheffield: Sexual Abuse Strategy Group.

Wyatt, G.E. Guthrie, D. and Notgrass, C.M. (1992), 'Differential effects of women's child sexual abuse and subsequent revictimization', *Journal of Counselling and Clinical Psychology*, 60, 167-173.

Wyatt, G.E. and Newcombe, M. (1990), 'Internal and external mediators of women's sexual abuse in childhood', *Journal of Counselling and Clinical Psychology*, 58, 758-767.

Chapter 13

Mental Health Promotion

Shulamit Ramon

Introduction

Mental health promotion is an old concept and approach, currently re-invented not only in the UK, but also globally.

This chapter will attempt to look at how it is defined, especially as distinct from public health and from other mental health activities, its links to psychosocial well being, and to the wider concepts of social inclusion, inequality, discrimination and its prevention, citizenship and social capital.

The issue of why it has re-gained greater centrality in governmental circles – and the assumed political significance of mental health promotion – will be focused upon, including the possibility of being used as another tool of social control within the *risk society*. We need to ask whether governmental commitment is yet another fashionable slogan, or is it accompanied by more substantial commitment to mental health promotion. Some of the core policies and measures associated with mental health promotion will be looked at in terms of what they promise, what they can fulfil, and what are the obstacles and opportunities which connect the promise to the realistic achievements of this policy, in particular in the context of vulnerable families, the workplace, and primary care.

Examples of good practice in a number of countries will be outlined and analysed.

Definitions, Conceptual Clarity, and Underpinning Ideologies

Mental health promotion has been constructed as a combination of two concepts: *mental health* and *health promotion.*

Mental health is usually given one of two definitions. Within medically oriented circles it is described as the absence of mental illness or disease, while within psychosocial approaches it is defined as mental wellbeing (Tudor, 1996).

The absence of an illness hinges on the professional decision as to the absence of any recognised symptoms of mental ill health, or – as is the case more often – whether existing symptoms amount to a syndrome (a chain of symptoms, assumed to co-exist and be dependent on each other), which would justify the attribution of an illness diagnosis. Thus the decision is not left to the person, but is assumed to be made on scientific grounds. The doubts pertaining to the validity and reliability of the psychiatric diagnostic system hold also for the decision that the person is mentally healthy.

Mental wellbeing is usually broken down to several dimensions to be achieved, or to act as indicators of an already achieved state. The dimensions include often a range from coping through social integration to self-actualisation and coherence (Jahoda, 1958; Tudor, 1996; Antonovsky, 1987). The list covers psychosocial relationships to self and to others, and to acting within a social world. The dimensions highlight the value of wellbeing not simply as a summary statement of where a person is, but also as a developmental and motivational factor.

Wellbeing contains a central subjective meaning element, one which does not exist in the definition of mental health as the absence of mental illness. It also incorporates:

- a social dimension in so far as feeling subjectively well is related to both being a member of a society and broadly accepting its definition of wellbeing, mental health, and of mental ill health
- satisfied basic health and psychological needs
- a degree of personal control over one's life (Ramon and Hart, 2003)
- a dimension of actualising one's potential (Ryan and Deci, 2001).

All of these features make mental wellbeing a much more complex concept than the absence of illness or disease, yet also a concept more difficult to observe and measure.

Traditional psychiatry rejects the validity of the subjective and the inter-subjective (social) dimensions of mental ill health in favour of its own assumed objective and universal framework, a framework it attempts to market in each society impacted by Western medicine.

The evidence for the existence of *universalised* mental ill health is paradoxical in so far as many of the symptoms of ill health are recognised as discrete behaviours beyond Western societies. However, their categorisation into mental illness symptoms or an illness category does not necessarily follow, and depends on the social significance attributed to these signs within a specific social system. Moreover, some of the signs are viewed as related to having exceptional personal qualities, perceived as a socially positive asset in societies in which the search for spirituality as a ritualised rite of passage and shamanism still exist (Erickson, 1951).

Furthermore, rates of recovery from severe mental illness are better in the developing world than they are in the developed world (Warner, 1985), even though the latter has at its disposal quantitatively more medication and of greater sophistication, psychotherapeutic methods, and rehabilitation programmes. This statistic is attributed to a lower level of stigma in the developing societies, associated with lower focus on material achievements, and a higher value attached to performing ordinary social roles unrelated to material achievements, such as being a family, neighbourhood and community member, than is the case in Western societies. Ironically we in Western societies lament the weakening of familial and communal bonds, see this weakness as an underlying cause for a number of personal and social ills such as addictions, homelessness, and mental illness, attempting to re-create these bonds (see the writings on Communitarianism for example, Etzioni, 1995). Yet on the whole we tend to ignore the connections highlighted above, as well as the contribution of conceptual and intervention frameworks which negate the very existence of these issues and connections, such as traditional psychiatry.

The rate of diagnosed minor mental illness is much lower in the developing world, a fact attributed to lack of social acceptance and recognition of these illness categories, and of being too preoccupied with survival issues to pay attention to mental distress.

Traditional psychiatry is neither able to account for the differences between the first and third worlds beyond claiming that less attention is paid to diagnosis in the latter, nor to learn the lessons from these differences in terms of their implications for the concepts of mental health and wellbeing as having inherent psychological and social dimensions at least as much as physical qualities, if not more.

Defining mental health as the absence of illness or disease makes us focus on identifying *risks* factors which would need to be eliminated or controlled to prevent the onset of illness. Thinking in risk *avoidance* terms appears to be widely accepted within both medicine and public health thinking.

It is also a negative definition in so far as it does not attribute any specific meaning or qualities to health apart from the negation of illness. This is an unsatisfactory definition from both lay and professional (scientific) perspectives, as it excludes further understanding of the concept. Most of us differentiate between not being hungry and enjoying our food, being dressed and being well dressed, feeling unwell, feeling OK and felling well, all of which are qualitative differences denied when health is defined as the absence of illness/disease.

Health promotion is defined as engaging in prevention, education, protection policies and methods in the field of health, aimed at improving the overall state of health of a population (Health Education Authority, 1997). It is a concept derived initially from public health, pragmatically utilised to embark on strategies and methods perceived as giving:

a.   at risk individuals and groups tools with which to improve their own health by increasing behaviours which enhance health and reduce vulnerability to a specific illness/disease and its debilitating symptoms
b.   tools for a more general healthy lifestyle (e.g. non-smoking, being physically fit through exercise and healthy foods).

The above puts the responsibility for one's health firmly within the duty and capacity of the individual, a belief which is questioned by those, including the author, who accept the impact of social factors on individuals as one which may at times render them unable and/or unwilling to take such a responsibility. For these dissenters the issue is how the interaction between individual and social responsibility is played out in a given society to enable, or disable, the promotion of health or mental health.

The critique of health promotion indicates that it tends to perpetuate paternalism and control of patients by health professionals, even when empowering and enabling aims are intended (Gilbert, 1995).

The inclusion of *social structural factors* within the equation of responsibilities for health promotion complicates not only the simple message, appealing or threatening as the case may be, of 'you can control your destiny'. It also implies the need for a more *holistic* understanding of the interaction between health and society, power relationships, and ultimately addressing the cause of social deprivation – a largely unpalatable political and professional message.

Once applied to mental health, the meaning of prevention, education and protection becomes less clear and the methods much less straightforward than in health promotion. This is in part due to the largely accepted understanding that the interaction between biological, psychological and social factors in mental health is much stronger at the etiological level, and therefore also at any of the facets just outlined. In addition, the early recognition of ill mental health is not a lay skill. This complexity does not lend itself to simple solutions or receipts.

Consequently, at the level of *prevention* alone we are looking at primary, secondary and tertiary prevention, each demanding a somewhat different understanding, policy, strategy, methods, and implementation mode. The complexity applies also to the different stakeholders who need to be addressed within mental health *education*; how they should be addressed, and the type of involvement we wish them to develop with mental health issues and people.

Protection is the least elaborated aspect within mental health promotion. Is it a synonym to primary prevention? Is it to be about developing resilience to adversity, or about promoting the factors, which support the development of mental health in any of its dimensions?

Working with children of parents experiencing mental health offers an interesting and useful example of an approach, which combines protection and prevention with the building up of resilience. Such projects can be found now in most Western countries. For example, the Netherlands has a national project for the last fifteen years with 50 community mental health centres in which preventative programmes are offered to children and their parents. Such programmes include home visiting interventions for depressed mothers and their babies, as well as the Beardslee psycho-educational programme family preventive programme (which also operates in the US, Finland, Belgium, Australia) (van Docsum, Bool and Hosman, 2002).

Diggins (2000) outlines a project based in an inner London area voluntary agency which works with the whole family as well as with any family member in need of support. For example, a mother with schizophrenia who has become isolated was encouraged to join a mothers and toddlers group, while her older child was in psychotherapy focused on his guilt feeling and isolation from the peer group.

Diggin's project and the Dutch innovative programme offer primary, secondary and tertiary prevention within the family system. The use of a variety of verbal and non-verbal techniques, such as drawing, caricatures, stories, and play in many of these projects adds to the challenge and the attraction.

The international Early Intervention in psychosis programme (McRory and Jackson, 1999) provides a useful example of a concerted effort to strengthen protective factors (e.g. providing psychotherapy, family work, education and vocational training) as well as reducing risk factors by the provision of medication and psycho-education which enables the person to identify early warning signs. This programme, however, does not work at the community level.

Ethical issues abound too. For example, should we advise people with mental illness not to have children because we have evidence which indicates that pregnancy is a crisis state for all women, and thus is more likely to be so for those already psychologically vulnerable? Or because more children of parents experiencing mental illness have such experiences themselves, in comparison to other children? Should we opt for a eugenic solution, namely state sponsored sterilisation of women who have mental illness, as was the case in the UK until the 1950s and in Sweden until the 1970s? Should we pay more positive attention to these children throughout their childhood? Should we tell women when they are put on psychiatric medication that this would reduce significantly their chances to conceive children?

It would seem that belief systems about human nature, social interaction, health and illness, dictate fashions in MHP.

Stages in the Recent Development of MHP within the Western World

The initial focus on prevention and promotion in mental health dates from the beginning of the 20th century and to the mental hygiene movement which originated in the US (Beers, 1908). The movement was closely connected to social engineering, increasing productivity in the workplace through fostering commitment to the workplace via the improvement of group cohesion. Some of its protagonists even saw a role for mental health in resolving international conflict. Some projects followed the initial enthusiasm. For example, Caplan's project on working with mothers of premature babies on reducing guilt, increasing bonding opportunities, and reducing the barriers to an active role for the mothers within the hospital wards outlined a new agenda for promoting mental health through the enhancement of protective factors (Caplan, 1961). Cumming and Cumming' (1957) work on reducing stigma by lay people towards those defined as mentally ill provides another example of this period, where educational methods were used to change such attitudes, without much success.

The establishment in the UK of therapeutic communities for traumatised soldiers during the 2nd World War can be seen as a tertiary prevention and health education programme in one (Rapaport, 1960). The communities enabled soldiers, their commanding officers, the army, and the involved public (mainly their relatives and friends) to legitimise war trauma and reduce considerably the stigma attached to it, as well as to stop the routine authorised shooting of such soldiers as deserters which was the official British army policy in the 1st World War. It offered these soldiers much needed therapeutic approach within the most democratic environment British psychiatry had had, thus marrying an individualistic and collectivistic approach. It also educated the army, mental health professionals, and the relatives that a war can trigger acute mental distress from which the majority can recover, with the due support they deserved. However, the contribution of this innovative programme to resolving international conflict was non-existent

The de-institutionalisation project which took place in the US, UK, Italy, Canada, New Zealand and Australia from the 1960s onwards provides a unique example of international comparison of tertiary prevention, paralleled only by the freeing of the mentally ill from their chains in the early 19th century, a truly heroic act of risk taking at that time. However, it is worth remembering that that policy ended by the adoption of large-scale psychiatric institutions, the very ones de-institutionalisation has/is dismantling. Some of the current fears expressed about de-institutionalisation are clearly echoing the late 19th and early 20th century beliefs in the need to re-segregate the mentally ill for their own sake and for the sake of the rest of us.

The message that the severely mentally ill can live in the community, and that the concrete structure in which they were contained (the hospital) is obsolete, has been a powerful one. The *visibility* of a group of people who have been hitherto segregated from sight, let alone touch and shared activity, used as a morality spectacle from the enlightenment period to the end of the Victorian era Bedlam (Porter, 2002), has dramatically shifted the grounds, by enabling them and us to re-discover their humanity.

For example, *L'una e l'altra* is a centre for women with and without mental health problems based in a renovated part of the old psychiatric hospital of Trieste, on the Adriatic coast of Italy and its border with Croatia and Slovenia. Most of the women experiencing mental health difficulties were long term patients in the institution.

The title is a play of words – the moon and its reflection, or one *is* the other in its female conjugation. The centre reflects the belief that fostering the shared interest of women as women can overcome the division introduced by mental ill health, levels of education and professionalism, age and ethnicity. The activities are decided by the participants, and vary from the political to the body beautiful, through attention to mental and physical health, poetry and theatre. Its members organised and participated in demonstrations for peace in Yugoslavia, debates on the origins of domestic violence and how to overcome it, as well as reading events on feminist literature and flower arrangement sessions.

The verdict as to whether the social inclusion of people with long term mental illness is an achievable objective beyond the trap of mini-institutionalisation in the community and the increasing incarceration in secure units of different descriptions which cater for the risk society agenda, remains to be reached. There are many powerful examples of such an inclusion by ex-patients who are now contributing positively to society in a variety of ways, from holding responsible jobs to running user-led projects (Sedley, 2000).

Wallcraft's chapter on *recovery* in this volume highlights that the agenda has moved on towards the end of the 20th century from rehabilitation to recovery for this high at risk population. Among other things, it outlines that it is possible to live with mental illness and yet lead a fulfilling life.

Recovery posits an interesting issue for mental health promotion, by encapsulating its different aspects of prevention, protection, and education simultaneously.

The end of the 20th century also marks the return of mental health promotion as part of the policy agenda for nation states mental health systems and beyond. Australia, the European Community, the four countries of the UK, and the WHO all see a prominent role for mental health promotion locally and internationally. The return can be understood in part as the outcome of the partial move away from the focus on people with long term mental illness to those with short term, usually minor, mental distress, who are the majority of sufferers and users of mental health and general health and social care systems, and who are predicted to multiple in number in the first two decades of the 21st century (Lehtinen *et al.*, 1997; Herman, 2001). We do have adequate methods of responding to their distress (Churchill *et al.*, 1998), but given the scale of the problem and its likely impact on economic productivity and family relationships it would be much better to nip it in the bud. However, these adequate response methods do not tackle the *underlying cause* of the increased rate, which seem to relate to the high level of uncertainty of the postmodern world, especially for otherwise vulnerable individuals.

The return to an active MHP agenda can also be understood as a result of the disappointment with the demonstrable limits of medical and psychological intervention methods, and the re-realisation of the need to use an all-system approach, which includes paying attention to social factors too. While not wanting to change the accepted social system of production – capitalism – the wish by official bodies to reduce the impact of its 'excesses' or 'weaknesses' which lead to social deprivation and inequality, and inevitably to the social exclusion of those thus impacted, resurfaces at the point in time in which the system goes through yet another fundamental change. Globalisation and computerisation of modes of production are such two changes we are facing presently.

The global effect of local political, and often violent conflict, has further demonstrated the impact of trauma caused through such a context on both combatant and non-combatant local people (Wolf and Mosnaim, 1990). The violent conflicts we are witnessing in many parts of the world for the last decade (e.g. Algeria, Chechnya, Columbia, Indonesia, The Middle East, Rwanda, Yugoslavia) affected whole populations. Becoming an internally displaced person is only mildly better than becoming an externally displaced person for the thousands of people who had to leave their homes, occupations, relatives and friends, for the sake of the unknown, even if physically safer, environment. Janet Williams' chapter in this volume on Trauma highlights the analysis of these situations and the appropriate interventions, which can support people who become their unwitting victims. Only a minority exhibits the symptoms of PTSD, while the majority gets on with the task of re-building their lives. Mental health promotion is of relevance to both the minority identified as being mentally ill and the majority which is sufficiently resilient not to demonstrate PTSD but which is affected in a number of other ways, such as lacking in optimism and self-confidence, giving up their dreams for self-fulfilment, adopting alienation, mistrust, exploitation, and cynicism as their main coping strategies, or living with consuming hatred of the other national group, waiting for the next moment of violent revenge to come.

Formal mental health promotion policies and strategies can support specific groups of victims and their helpers. Yet MHP per se can do little to change such perspectives. However, strategies focused on *re-building* shattered communities can slowly enable members of each community to find a new anchor and a renewed dialogue with the other group which has been both the enemy and contributing neighbours. Northern Ireland (Hargie and Dixon, 2004) has a number of such examples, in which victims of sectarian violence are helped individually to the point of stopping to be a victim, side by side with supporting their communities to re-build their economic, leadership, and solidarity bases. Experience has shown that it is only when these bases have been re-built that the dialogue with the other community can began without an overarching need for revenge.

Evidence and its Value

The evidence we have on the success of primary prevention is at best patchy (Mentality, 2000a). This is hardly surprising given the level of complexity and the number of factors any such strategy has to entail. Let us look at one of the more daring examples of tackling primary prevention in the UK, namely Sure Start (www.surestart.gov.uk). Sure Start is the flagship preventative programme of New Labour, which came into being soon after Labour came back into power in 1997 after 18 years out of government. Influenced by the American Head Start programme of the 1960s and 1970s, but also introducing its own original features, Sure Start is aimed at supporting and working with vulnerable families of children below four years of age at any needed facet to prevent the creation and accumulation of social and psychological (i.e. psychosocial) deprivation by the parents, siblings and the young children themselves, to ensure a future free of such vulnerabilities.

Vulnerabilities can be material (state of housing), financial (level of income), educational (level of parental education, formal and informal educational opportunities for the children), social (newcomers immigrant families, integrating white and non-white families), psychological (poor bonding, poor martial relationships), physical (domestic violence, physical handicap, chronic illness of either parents or children), legal (being asylum seekers, a parent who has offended, children in breach of the law, having an employer who does not follow the employment law).

Where Does Such a Programme Start? Where Should it End?

Local Sure Start programmes were given some autonomy in choosing their priorities from this wide ranging menu, but had to demonstrate outcomes within one year. Most of these outcomes are in reality *process* outcomes, namely indicators of the number of people involved, the activities in which they participate, and modes of participation. Some activities are short-lived either because they were planned in this way or because they did not work out as planned. For example, a women's group focused on domestic violence has been planned to last for six meetings, on the assumption that the local women likely to participate in it would not be able to come for a longer period. Yet six meetings are insufficient to move beyond scratching the surface of this highly emotive and sensitive issue. However, the success of the first round on domestic violence has illustrated to the organisers the importance of the issue and the readiness of some local women to commit themselves to a group focused on it, even if it meant risking a journey of six flights of stairs on an estate in which lifts are often stuck, with some small children and children's buggies in toe. The group recruited women from a specific ethnic minority and not from others or from the local white majority population. This provided another important lesson, namely that not all issues can be safely discussed by all women. It was possible to create a wider collaboration around issues such as a nursery for children with special needs; yet it was nearly impossible to recruit men to any group, including unemployed men, unless they were given position of power and/or prestige.

Women and men's gainful employment emerged as the key for their children's future from their perspective, even though they understood that educational opportunities for the children are not less important. Yet the pursuit of adults' gainful employment is not recognised as a priority issue within the programme, because of its focus on parenting and young children, and support for employment is provided as a sideline derived from the wish to follow individuals' agendas. A working mother has less time and energy to give to her children, yet the evidence highlights that children of working mothers – girls (daughters) in particular – are more likely to do better regards their future employment then children of mothers who opted to be housewives and full-time mothers.

The Place of Governmental Policy

The seriousness of governmental intentions towards meeting a MHP agenda can be judged by the dedicated (ring-fenced) funding given to it, as well as by how well integrated is this agenda into the agenda of the various systems which are interwoven within it, to include not only mental health services, but also systems responsible for primary care, education, employment, criminal justice and immigration. In the UK MHP has become part of the official mental health policy only in 1999 (see Standard 1 in The National Framework for Mental Health, published by the Department of Health, 1999). Thus far each area health authority had to plan an area implementation policy by the end of 2001. Authorities varied considerably in the degree of effort, stakeholders' participation, and creativity which went into this phase, facilitated nationally by a number of government sponsored position and evidence papers (Mentality, 2000b). The fact that the MHP national lead group consisted of a very small unit within the Department of Health conveyed the message of the limited importance of the project, at least at that stage.

The published plans differed in scope and focus, from those which centred only on tertiary prevention, to those which focused mainly on primary prevention. Most staff working in secondary services did not see themselves involved in the implementation of these plans, arguing that they were too busy with implementing governmental demands to do with mental illness targets.

Those already working in MHP projects were keen to continue to do so, but felt very much left to their own devices, especially as projects were funded for a limited period of time.

Four years later some MHP objectives have become an integral part of the newly created National Institute of Mental Health (NIMH) for England only which has a brief for innovation in mental health services. For example, its *social inclusion* agenda has entailed the appointment of social inclusion and wider participation fellows whose role is to research the availability of socially inclusionary services and projects in the fields of education, employment, leisure, housing, as the first step towards ensuring that users of mental health services have adequate access to these services. At this stage the focus of the social inclusion aspect is on MHP at the level of secondary and tertiary prevention.

Promoting mental wellbeing in the workplace is recognised as an important issue within each national economy, given the number of productivity days lost each year due to mental distress and illness (Wainwright and Calnan, 2002). It is also mentioned as a central issue in each updated national MHP plan, and has attracted research on its causes and many proposals and projects on reducing the burden by employees and employing organisations. (Morrow *et al.*, 2002) The issue is complex, due to the contribution of both personalised and organisational underlying factors. The evidence pertaining to the success of the various initiatives is not surprisingly inconclusive, given this complexity, even though most workers suffering from mental distress tend to experience minor difficulties, which can be resolved to the satisfaction of both employees and employers within a relatively short time and effort. Nevertheless, and despite the fact that this issue has been looked at from the inception of MHP, employers' and managers' attitudes towards employees experiencing mental distress continue to be negative and accusatory. Most organisations do not have effective policies which support employees at the crucial stages of onset of problems and return to work; most employees are sure that admitting to having mental health problems will damage their career, and most managers continue to believe that such employees are 'weaklings', rather than it is the combination of organisational culture and individual vulnerabilities which need to be tackled.

Thus the case of promoting mental wellbeing in the workplace highlights the impact of public attitudes towards mental illness and health, as well as the fine balance between experiencing stress and intolerable stress, the centrality of feeling in control as the key to not experiencing stress as intolerable, and the need to believe that management really cares about the objectives of the organisation and about its employees. My own research on this issue (Ramon and Hart, 2003; Beckwith and Munn-Giddings, 2003; Ramon and Morris, 2004) focused on applying participatory strategy principles by engaging employees in a health trust and a social services department in analysing the factors associated with a high level of stress and mental distress, and the solutions which will work to enable workers to live with it, without becoming unable to function properly in the workplace. The factors which came high as leading to stress included a poor physical environment, but most of them had to do with poor communication between management and employees, not being in control in the job, and feeling unvalued. Anonymous questionnaire data corroborated these findings. While most workers experienced high levels of stress they also had their own support systems, mainly outside of the working environment. The minority who did not have such a support sub-system were likely to find stress intolerable and likely to develop mental distress.

Mental health promotion is a life cycle issue, affecting each of us, far beyond mental illness. We have a long way to go before its complexity is better understood and before it will be taken with the seriousness it deserves by most social institutions.

References

Antonovsky, A. (1987), *Unravelling the Mystery of Health: How People Manage Stress and Stay Well*, Jossey Bass, San Francisco.

Beers, C. (1980), *A Mind That Found Itself*, Longmans, New York.

Beckwith, D. and Munn-Giddings, C. (2003), 'Self-help/mutual aid in promoting mental health at work', *Journal of Mental Health Promotion*, 2, 4, 14-25.

Caplan, G. (1961), *An Approach to Community Mental Health*, Grune and Stratton, New York.

Churchill, R., Wesseley, S. and Lewis, G. (1998), 'A systematic review and meta-analysis of the effects of combining pharmacotherapy and psychotherapy for the treatment of depression', *The Cochrane Library*, Oxford Update Software.

Cumming, E. and Cumming, J. (1957), *Closed Ranks: An Experiment in Mental Health Education*, Harvard University Press, Cambridge MA.

Diggins, M. (2000), 'Innovation as a Way of Professional Life: The Building Bridges Project for Parents-users of Mental Health services and their Children', in: Ramon, S. (ed.), *A Stakeholder's Approach to Innovation in Mental Health Services: A Reader for the 21st Century*, Pavilion Publishing, Brighton, 77-94.

Department of Health (1999), *The National Framework for Mental Health: Standards and Models*, HMSO, London.

Erickson, E. (1951), *Childhood and Society*, Basic Books, New York.

Etzioni, A. (1995), *The Spirit of Community: Rights, Responsibilities and the Communitarian Agenda*, Fontana Press, Glasgow.

Gilbert, T. (1995), 'Nursing: Empowerment and the problem of power', *Advanced Nursing*, 16, 354-361.

Health Education Authority (1997), *Mental Health Promotion*, HEA, London.

Hargie, O. and Dixon, D. (2004), *Researching The Troubles: Social Sciences Perspective on the Northern Ireland Conflict*, Mainstream Publishing, Edinburgh.

Herman, H. (2001), 'The need for mental health promotion', *Australian and New Zealand Journal of Psychiatry*, 35, 709-715.

Jahoda, M. (1958), *Current Positive Mental Health*, Basic Books, New York.

Lehtinen, V., Rijkonen, E. and Lahtinen, E. (1997), *Promotion of Mental Health and the European Agenda*, National Research and Development centre for Welfare and Health, STAKES, Helsinki.

McRory, P. and Jackson, H. (1999), *The Recognition and Management of Early Psychosis: A Preventive Approach*, Cambridge University Press, Cambridge.

Mentality (2000a), Briefing paper on the Evidence Base for the White Paper on Mental Health, Mentality, London.

Mentality (2000b), *Making It Happen*, Department of Health, London.

Morrow, L., Verins, I. and Willis, E. (eds) (2002), *Mental Health and Work*, Commonwealth of Australia, Bedford Park.

Porter, R. (2002), *Madness: A Brief History*, Oxford University Press.

Ramon, S. Hart, C. (2003), 'Promoting mental wellbeing in the workplace: A British Case', *International Journal of Mental Health*, 5, 2, 37-44.

Ramon, S. and Morris, L. (2004), 'Responding to Stress and mental distress in social services: Applying a participatory strategy', forthcoming, *Research, Planning and Policy Journal*.

Rapaport, R. (1960), *Community as Doctor*, Tavistock, London.

Ryan, R. and Deci, E. (2001), 'On happiness and human potentials: A review of research on hedonic and eudaimanic wellbeing', *Annual Review of Psychology*, 52, 141-166.

Sedley, B. (2000), Why Change Anything?, in: Ramon, S. (ed.), *A Stakeholder's Approach of Innovation in Mental Health Services: A Reader for the 21st Century*, Pavilion Publishing, Brighton, 47-59.

Tudor, K. (1996), *Mental Health Promotion: Paradigms and Practice, Routledge*, London.

Van Doesum, K., Bool, M. and Hosman, C. (2002), 'Training of professionals for the benefit of the children of mentally ill parents', 2nd World Congress of the Promotion of Mental Health, London, 11-12 September.

Wainwright, D. and Calnan, M. (2002), *Work Stress: The Making of a Modern Epidemic*, Open University Press, Buckingham.

Warner, R. (1985), *Recovery from Schizophrenia*, Routledge, London.

Wolf, M.E. and Mosnaim, A.D. (eds) (1990), *Posttraumatic Stress Disorder: Etiology, Phenomenology, and Treatment*, American Psychiatric Press, Washington DC.

Chapter 14

Re-introducing the Psychosocial in Training, Education and Research

Julia Jones and Catherine Gamble

Introduction

Over the last decade, innovations in treatment and intervention strategies, incorporating psychological and social perspectives alongside biological approaches, have reformed the way that people with severe and enduring mental health problems are cared for. The increasing use of psychosocial interventions (PSI) as a multidisciplinary approach has brought with it a more holistic understanding of strategies that can be used to manage some of the most disabling symptoms of illnesses, such as schizophrenia and bi-polar disorder. It is now widely accepted that better outcomes can be achieved when medication alone is not used as the panacea for treating every symptom or behaviour experienced. A more holistic approach, which recognises environmental, psychological and biological vulnerabilities, incorporating people's social contexts and their relationships with significant others, is now heralded as the way forward.

This chapter provides an overview of the emergence of psychosocial interventions as a way of treating and working with people who have severe and enduring mental health problems, and their carers (defined in this chapter as all those significant individuals who support the service user). The background and philosophy behind the research, education, training and development of PSI is addressed, before moving on to focus on its clinical aspects, through the use of a case scenario. This encapsulates the key components of the PSI approach and provides examples of how to overcome potential or actual barriers regarding the implementation of this approach.

Background

Since the 1980s, new directions in psychosocial approaches have developed through the findings of research studies that suggest that 'ambient stress', combined with life events and unsupportive environments, may trigger onset or relapse in schizophrenia (Neuchterlein and Dawson, 1984; Leff and Vaughn, 1985; Zubin and Spring, 1977). These inaugural studies, in combination with the outcomes from assertive community treatment trials (Marks *et al.*, 1994), led to the development of a

Psychosocial Interventions training programme, initially for community psychiatric nurses (CPNs) (Gamble, 1995). This programme, called the Thorn Initiative, sought to expand nurses' knowledge, enhance their skills, challenge pessimistic assumptions held about schizophrenia and its prognosis and thereby reduce professionals' reliance on psychotropic medication and hospital admissions to manage symptoms.

A number of research studies (Brooker *et al.*, 1994; Lancashire *et al.*, 1997; Leff *et al.*, 2001) have provided a growing body of evidence of favourable outcomes for users and carers from the training of nurses, CPNs, in psychosocial approaches. The positive outcomes from these educational programmes have stimulated national recognition that training, combined with user and carer involvement in curriculum development and teaching activities, is the key to developing collaborative working relationships, embracing new service concepts and enhancing care provision. This approach differs from any previous training because it comprehensively incorporates all the above, as well as measuring the impact of the training upon the health and social functioning of the service users with whom the nurses, undergoing the training, are working with (Gamble, 1997).

There are now at least 75 PSI training courses, located mainly in England, that range from short courses and diplomas to Master's level (Brooker *et al.*, 2003). Training now involves all members of the multidisciplinary team, not just nurses, and is responsive to intervention advances, such as early intervention, psychopharmacology, dual diagnosis and the promotion of social inclusion. The training does not simply focus upon biological theories of the nature and cause of mental illness and treating it with medication alone; the training incorporates cultural, psychological and social models of health so that a more comprehensive appraisal of people's needs and strengths can be met. The training also focuses upon the importance of recovery and helping service users through individualised, tailor made self-help methods, such as the normalisation of experiences, spirituality and complementary therapies, with the underlying aim that the users of mental health services, with whom the trainees work, will feel more empowered, valued and able to function within society.

However training is only the beginning of the process; the training programmes seek to ensure that the philosophy of inclusion and interventions taught are implemented in clinical practice. Therefore, unlike many other training or academic courses, strong links are established prior to, during and post training with clinical supervisors, service leaders and managers. In addition, the courses are designed to promote user involvement by incorporating the expertise of users and carers into curriculum development, teaching and supervision teams, with the aim of reducing exclusivity and endorsing the philosophy that knowledge and expertise is shared, both during and beyond training.

The Theoretical Underpinnings of PSI: Expressed Emotion and the Stress-vulnerability Model

The development of psychosocial interventions emerged from the seminal work of Brown, Birley and Wing (1972) which identified Expressed Emotion (EE) within family settings as a factor that influences the frequency of relapse in people suffering from schizophrenia. Expressed Emotion (EE) refers to response characteristics of family members living with individuals with schizophrenia. Research has indicated that high EE responses, such as critical, hostile or emotional over-involvement with the relative with schizophrenia, has a negative impact on the occurrence of relapse (Leff and Vaughn, 1985).

During the same time period, influential stress-vulnerability models were emerging (Zubin and Spring, 1977; Neuchterlein and Dawson, 1984), drawing attention to the importance of social and environmental factors, in particular 'ambient stress', on the course and prognosis of schizophrenia. According to these models, symptoms are viewed as the product of life stressors and the person's predisposition to cope with that stress in combination with their illness. Understanding this relationship, within the context of the developing work on family intervention (discussed later in this chapter), has assisted with the development of broad models of psychosocial educational programmes (Barrowclough and Tarrier, 1992; Kuipers, *et al.*, 1992; Falloon and Graham-Hole, 1994).

Definition of Psychosocial Interventions

Unfortunately there is no commonly agreed single definition of psychosocial interventions. A useful definition, that we will use as the 'working definition' of PSI for this chapter, comes from the 'Avoiding the Washout' document (Repper and Brooker, 2002), which states that:

> Psychosocial interventions has become a term that can best be understood as an ideological and political force within contemporary mental health practice that seeks to challenge a dominant non-recovery approach to working with psychosis. It supports the vision that an integrated approach to aid the process of self discovery is a basic human right of people who experience psychosis and their carers. This leads to the premise that the mental health workforce possesses positive attitudes, up to date knowledge and a wide range of skills to help individuals and carers improve the quality of their lives (p. 42).

Core Components of Current PSI Training Courses

This section presents the key components of PSI currently taught in the UK.

1) Outcome Orientated Assessment

Conducting a systematic assessment is an integral part of psychosocial interventions. According to Gamble and Brennan (2000a) the areas of an individual's life that should be included in an assessment include: risk; physical and mental health status; social needs and functioning; symptoms and coping skills; quality of life and its effects on others; housing and money; social support; medicine and its effects; and work skills and meaningful daily activity. Some authors advocate the use of the semi-structured interview as a good way to begin the assessment, to establish rapport with an individual and enable them to 'tell their story' in their own words and identify their own goals (Clinton and Nelson, 1996; Fox and Conroy, 2000). This interview can then be supplemented with more focused assessment tools, designed to identify specific information that may emerge from the initial interview (Fox and Conroy, 2000).

Until recently, the routine use of standardised assessment tools (see Gamble and Brennan, 2000a) has not been actively valued by practitioners, as they have generally been perceived as burdensome paperwork that can prevent therapeutic alliances being developed. Yet findings from a large scale study from the service user perspective (Rose, 2001), identified that 17-36 per cent of clients felt professionals had not assessed their needs properly, and an even higher proportion of them (30-79 per cent) reported that their strengths and abilities had not been taken into account. This finding supports the role of a structured and systematic assessment process, using both qualitative and quantitative methods, as required, to conduct a comprehensive assessment of users' and carers' needs.

2) Medication Management

The evaluation of the efficacy and tolerance of medication is clearly an important component of comprehensive mental health care. However, many service users consistently express their concerns regarding the negative side effects of medication (NSF, MDF and Mind, 2001, 2002) that can significantly affect users' quality of life and discourage them from taking their medication consistently (Sin and Gamble, 2003). Whilst many users do take an active role in negotiating their medication regimes, doctors (and now also some nurses) hold the power and knowledge to prescribe, and this unequal relationship can make some users feel powerless and without a voice in the treatment process (Carrick *et al.*, 2004). The purpose of providing training to professionals in medication management is to educate and inform them about the role of pharmacology in the treatment of serious mental illness and to enable them to work more effectively with their clients with regard to providing information, supporting and working *with* them, and their carers, in the management of medication.

Recent research studies have followed the progress of nurses who have undertaken training in medication management and show that these nurses improve in both their knowledge and clinical skills (Gray *et al.*, 2001; Gray *et al.*, 2003). These studies also demonstrate that such training benefits both professionals' and users' understanding of the role of medication within the recovery process, as well as seeing a positive improvement in users' symptoms. It is clear that to make these findings more inclusive, further research needs to be conducted across the mental health disciplines and to continue to evaluate users' experiences of taking medication (e.g. Faulkner and Layzell, 2000; Carrick *et al.*, 2004).

3) Psychological Management of Psychosis and Early Intervention

Research has identified a variety of strategies for professionals and their clients, working within a therapeutic relationship, to help people cope with hearing voices and having strange, worrying beliefs (Mills, 2000). The seminal work of Roome and Esher (1993) has played an important role; their epidemiological research identified that many 'mentally healthy' people in western society hear voices and live very successful lives without psychiatric intervention. They achieve this by not only retaining their own sense of identity in their dealings with their voices, but by accepting and working with their experiences. Roome and Esher (1993) and others (Bentall, 2003) have challenged the notion that the first therapeutic response should be to reach for a prescription pad to relieve suffering, as this action is considered to impede the search for a solution and increase the chance of recurrence (Roome and Esher, 2000). For people who hear voices, this new way of thinking has contributed to greater acceptance and support to find ways of coping with their voices, other than medication (Baker, 2003).

The impact of this development on training is a new focus on treatments that aim to enhance individual coping strategies and review the impact the voice hearing experience has upon a person and those around them (Mills, 2000). Training now involves how to conduct an initial comprehensive assessment of the user's psychotic experiences, so that specific interventions can then be used appropriately. Further techniques taught include: modifying delusional beliefs, using Socratic questioning (a particular questioning style, see Fowler Garety and Kuipers, 1995: 98); non confrontational reality testing; decreasing the impact of hallucinations; using thought stopping; verbal challenging; and belief modification.

Psychosis tends to emerge during the mid to late teenage years and early twenties, at a crucial developmental stage for young people. There is a growing body of research evidence that suggests that when mental health services are offered early, that are appropriate and sensitive to the distinctive needs of an individual, then there is a reduction of long-term problems and a better chance of recovery for young people (Sainsbury Centre for Mental Health, 2003). The early intervention approach involves early signs monitoring to prevent relapse, drawing upon the principles of cognitive behavioural therapy (CBT). The purpose of the approach is to help users and their carers, supported by professionals, to develop their understanding of what exacerbates relapse and the signs that indicate it.

Research evidence regarding the effectiveness of this approach is still in its infancy, and has focused primarily on people with a diagnosis of schizophrenia, but existing studies suggest that early intervention can reduce incidents of relapse as well as length of stay in hospital (Birchwood, 1996). This approach has also been found to be useful for those with other disorders, such as Bi-polar, where psycho-educational techniques are used to help users to monitor and pre-empt relapse and extend length of time between manic episodes (Perry *et al.*, 1999). These educational approaches provide a unique learning, for professionals, users and carers, to share expertise in understanding the social and environmental factors that can trigger relapse vulnerability (Birchwood *et al.*, 2000; Sainsbury Centre for Mental Health, 2003; Initiative to Reduce the Impact of Schizophrenia website).

Family Assessment of Needs and Intervention

Family interventions are based on broad psycho-educational and/or behavioural approaches that have been derived from research-based studies into Expressed Emotion, as described earlier in the chapter. There are currently three main models of family intervention that are practiced in the UK:

- *Cognitive behaviour intervention* (Barrowclough and Tarrier, 1992), a cognitive and behavioural approach to working collaboratively with users and carers, which includes: the initial assessment of users' and carers' needs; providing psycho-education for carers; stress management and coping strategies; dealing with violence and suicide risk; how to engage and maintain everyone's involvement
- *Family work for schizophrenia* (Kuipers *et al.*, 1992), combines psychotherapeutic principles with problem solving approaches and includes: assessment of the user and their family members; engaging the family; improving communication; identification of stressors; setting realistic goals; dealing with emotional issues (e.g. anger, conflict, rejection); dealing with over-involvement; employment, cultural and special issues (e.g. substance abuse, suicide, incest)
- *Behavioural Family Therapy* (Falloon and Graham-Hole, 1994) that assesses all family members' needs and then implements behavioural-type learning and problem-solving, via specific behavioural tasks, which incorporate learning how to listen, praise, be assertive and make positive requests

The main conclusions of existing studies into the effectiveness of family intervention are that these approaches, when combined with medication, may decrease frequency of relapse, can encourage compliance with medication and may improve social impairment and the levels of EE found in families (Pharoah *et al.*, 2003). This approach has not only been used with family members; staff in community residential facilities have also benefited from being taught components of family intervention (Willets and Leff, 1997). Regarding the usefulness of this approach from the carer perspective, one study of carers' experiences of family intervention reported positive impacts of the intervention to include: an increased knowledge about, and understanding of, their relative's illness; feeling more supported, both socially and emotionally; a greater understanding and tolerance of their relative's behaviour; and improved communication between family members (Budd and Hughes, 1997).

Collaborative Case Management and the Care Programme Approach (CPA)

Case management is a model of mental health care aimed specifically at people with severe and enduring mental health problems, with the objective to ensure that service users are: 'provided with whatever services they need in a co-ordinated, effective, and efficient manner' (Intagliata, 1982: 657). The case management approach was first developed in the USA and has subsequently been adopted and adapted in other countries. There are three main models of case management practiced in the UK: *Clinical case management* (Kanter, 1989); *The strengths model* (Rapp, 1998); and the *assertive community treatment model (ACT)*, developed from the research work of Stein and Test (1980) in the US. The research evidence regarding the effectiveness of these different models is conflicting (Mueser, 1998; Simpson *et al.*, 2003a). However, studies from a user perspective suggest that it is the quality of the relationship between the user and professional, rather than the mode of delivery, that is most relevant to the success of case management (Beeforth *et al.*, 1994; Repper *et al.*, 1994).

The care programme approach (CPA) is based upon the general case management approach, as developed in the US, and was introduced in England as national mental health policy in 1991 (Department of Health, 1990). The aim of CPA was to improve the coordination of community care for people with severe mental health problems. However, despite many revisions and reforms since 1991 the CPA is still not considered to be effective at the national level, with considerable variation in its operation (Scheider *et al.*, 1999; Social Services Inspectorate, 1999). Furthermore, some studies have reported that for many service users and carers, CPA remains relatively invisible or ineffectual (Rose, 2001; Simpson, 2003b).

Putting Research, Education and Training in PSI into Practice

So far, we have described the current research, education and training in the field of psychosocial interventions. However, training is only the beginning of a long learning process, both for mental health professionals, users, carers, health and social care organisations. In this section, we aim to illustrate the potential impact of the research, education and training around PSI, but also the continued complexities of implementation in 'real life' clinical practice, through a fictional case scenario.

Case Scenario

James, aged 20, dropped out of university and returned to live with his parents. He was reluctant to explain his behaviour but eventually disclosed that he thought his degree course in chemistry was too basic and that he would achieve more studying at home. Over the next two years James became increasingly isolative. His family fluctuated from being merely bemused by his odd behaviour to becoming very concerned that his whole persona was changing. Perceiving that his behaviour to be more then just wilfulness on James part, his mother managed to persuade him to visit the GP. The meeting raised the GP's concerns, so he referred James to the local psychiatric hospital. James refused to attend. He reassured his parents that he would socialise more and signed up for a local college course and so their immediate concerns subsided. However, James began to pick arguments with other students, he was disruptive in class and his attendance became erratic. At the same time James reported being followed home by 'dark spirited' free masons who were infiltrating the college.

James' non-attendance at the psychiatric hospital was reviewed by the community mental health team, who were concerned by the GP's report. One member of the team contacted James, who after some gentle persuasion agreed to be visited at home. The initial visit highlighted that James was clearly experiencing psychotic symptoms; he intermittently paced around the room, was highly distractible and mumbled to himself whilst his parents tried to fill in the information gaps and explain the family's concerns and worries. However, James did talk about how the free masons were destroying his life and he asked if anything could be done to get rid of them.

This was deemed as a window of opportunity to engage James and support his bewildered family. A subsequent clinical review meeting identified that the care programme should incorporate:

a)   An ongoing assessment to monitor and manage James' needs, social functioning and symptoms
b)   Monitoring and managing his antipsychotic medication
c)   A psycho-educational component that would help James learn the skills to cope with hearing voices, and to challenge and modify his beliefs about his psychotic experiences, as and when necessary
d)   A relapse prevention plan, incorporating early warning signs and coping strategies
e)   A collaborative care package that would encompass all the above, and include James' family's needs with the view to developing a tailor made, supportive intervention that will introduce James and his family to the team and mental care system.

This scenario, up until this point, should see a comprehensive package of care being delivered to James and his family. However, it does not always work like this in practice. The following section discusses the initial actions that are taken by the team, with potential problems and barriers that may present themselves, and how these may be overcome.

The Process of Assessment

Previous assessments may have been carried out with James that have not been recorded and are therefore unknown to the team. This could potentially alienate James from the engagement process, as there is nothing worse than having to re-tell your story. Therefore the team needs to establish whether there have been previous assessments conducted. A process of systematic assessment should then be followed, using methods and tools that are appropriate, valid and reliable, sensitive to change and easy to follow and use. It is also important that James is asked to describe the things he wants to work towards, i.e. his goals. A structured process of assessment should then lead naturally on to intervention, with practitioners knowing what to do with the information that has been gathered.

It is crucial that any assessment is conducted in a collaborative way and that James and his family (and other significant others) do not feel that they are subjected to a series of assessments that are simple 'done' to them by professionals. Therefore the purpose of conducting assessments should be clearly explained to James and his family, with information from the assessment reported back in an appropriate and sensitive way. In addition, James and his family could be informed about self-assessment tools that assist people (users and carers) to make their own assessment, with the support from others, such as the CUES tool (Lelliott *et al.*, 2001) or the Avon Mental Health Measure (see: MIND website) that have been developed from the user and carer perspective. Such tools, for example, can help users and carers prepare for, and also take a prominent place in, care planning meetings (Turner, 2001).

In summary, James' team may wish to consider the following:

- Find out whether James has had previous assessments conducted by talking to James and his family, as well as James' GP
- Provide information to James and his family about the rationale for assessments, before conducting any
- Offer to support James and his family to conduct their own self-assessments, using tools such as CUES or the Avon Mental Health Measure
- In line with the concept of recovery, James' short, medium and long term life goals to be addressed and reviewed (Repper and Perkins, 2003). For example, James may wish to return to university. However, James may also be fearful of this, worried about the effects of stress and/or fear of other people's reaction to his condition. To help overcome potential fears and other obstacles, James' team could liaise with his university's welfare officers; research shows that when there is collaboration (with the student's permission) between health services and educational institutions, then a student's return to study is more likely to be successful (Leach, 2003)
- Helping James with practical things, such as income and benefits, housing, finding a part-time job or doing voluntary work, engaging in more social activities, etc.

Medication Management

James may have been prescribed medication that both his psychiatrist and GP are happy with, but James is not because he cannot cope with the side effects. It has been suggested that a successful response to medication can provide the necessary foundation for recovery (Francell, 2002), and that many users appreciate the benefits of appropriate medication and the lessening of symptoms (Rose, 2001). Nevertheless, people have different opinions about what is, and what is not, tolerable. For example, James may find the side effects more troublesome than his symptoms and in this case, it is important that the team respects and values James' views. These issues need to be addressed. Accordingly, James' team may wish to incorporate the following:

- Explore James past and current experiences of taking medication
- Encourage James to become an active participant in his treatment by providing information, options, listening, being consistent and understanding that medication is not the be all and end all (Francell, 2002)
- Ensure that team members working with James have a good knowledge and understanding of antipsychotic medication and the clinical skills to conduct the systematic assessment and management of adverse side effects that James may be experiencing, making changes to medication as required (Sin and Gamble, 2003)
- Elicit and review with James the direct and indirect benefits of taking medication. A subjective assessment tool, such as the Liverpool University Neuroleptic Side-Effect Rating Scale (LUNSERS) (Day *et al.*, 1995), may be helpful
- Use motivational interviewing techniques to explore James' hesitancy or ambivalence about changing to a life style that not only incorporates new methods of coping with his symptoms and experiences, but includes taking medication.

Psychological Management of Psychosis and Early Intervention

Interventions c) and d) make the assumption that James is prepared at this point to modify his beliefs about his psychotic experiences. This may not be the case and it should be acknowledged that James' particular experiences might affect his participation in any treatment. Team members need to acknowledge that integral to the psychosocial approach is the development of a therapeutic working relationship. James is just entering into the mental health system, therefore the development of a positive therapeutic, working alliance at this early stage is essential, as this can have a fundamental enduring effect upon his relationship with team members and services (Drury, 2000) as well as his potential for recovery (Sainsbury Centre for Mental Health, 2003). It is therefore important to gradually ease first onset clients into therapy (Chadwick, *et al.*, 1996). This often requires practitioners to be creative and flexible about the timing, frequency and whereabouts of where formal sessions are conducted (Mills, 2000).

These early sessions with James, conducted by a team member with CBT training, are augmented with a basic CBT framework that involves incorporating the ABC model (Activating events, Beliefs and Consequences, see Mills, 2000). Using this model, James is slowly encouraged to examine and record what sort of situations Activated or exacerbated the 'Free Masons' and the Beliefs he held about those ideas or thoughts. Over time, it is possible for James to begin to understand the emotional or behavioural Consequences that the Belief invoked. By understanding and utilising these principles, James sees improvements in his self-esteem and his ability to manage symptoms more effectively, his stress and anxiety reduce considerably and so does the amount of medication he needs.

However, the challenge for the team member who has been working with James is how to share the outcomes of the meetings with James with the rest of the clinical team and James' family. Not all team members agree with sharing information either between themselves, or with his family, about particular aspects of James psychotic experiences and the early warning signs that he has disclosed, because they fear it would breach confidentiality (Furlong and Leggart, 1996; Szmukler and Bloch, 1997). This situation can create problems directly for the team's collaborative working and indirectly, upon the coordination of care for James and his family.

In summary, the team could implement the following actions:

- James to be given information about, and involved in decisions regarding, the CBT that he is receiving. For example, when, where and how often the sessions take place
- Individual meetings to be held with James, to review what he wishes to discuss with his family; recent research, conducted by users and carers, has shown that users and carers can have different opinions regarding the sharing of information about treatment (Allam *et al.*, 2004)
- Team members to review their own understanding of confidentiality, ideally in conjunction with local users and carer groups
- Team members to ensure they are all working to the same agenda, with a focus on their abilities to promote the principles of recovery and to implement evidence-based approaches
- James and his family to be given information and contact details for self-help groups for people who hear voices, such as the Hearing Voices Network (www.hearing-voices.org).

Family Assessment of Needs and Intervention

Some families initially deal with the family member's presenting problems by setting behavioural limits, emotionally distancing themselves from the situation and/or relying on religious beliefs. Others, in an attempt to deal with their own sadness, anger, shame, guilt, and resentment, avoid conflict and confrontation when a loved one is diagnosed with a psychotic disorder (Teschinsky, 2000). Judgements about how families are coping can easily be made if team members are not trained and/or responsive to such coping styles. For example, team members may want to immediately implement a structured family intervention programme, consisting of regular meetings and follow-ups with James and his parents, as members of the team have been trained in this and are enthusiastic about its potential impact.

However, James' mother feels uneasy about this suggestion, as no-one has offered help before and she feels she has coped well over the last two years. When these feelings are not initially identified within the assessment process, and are subsequently ignored by the team, James' mother feels that her views have been dismissed and she refuses to formally participate. However, she does agree to see a team member at her home, after she finishes work, to discuss the issue further. Unfortunately, the community mental health team does not operate out-of-hours home visits, when she is available. To promote engagement and inclusion, there is clearly a need to address current rigid service structures so that individual needs and requests can be addressed at both clinical and organisational levels.

In summary, the following actions should be addressed by the team (and the wider organisation):

- It should not be assumed by the team that the family would want to participate in family intervention. Many families are initially suspicious when family work is suggested and may often refuse to participate. This should not be perceived as a rejection by the team and the invitation should be left open and contact maintained. If families agree to hear more, team members should take time to listen, provide information, reflect upon the family's experiences of service provision, ascertain what can be learnt and subsequently offer a programme of care, based upon the assessed needs of the family (Gamble and Brennan, 2000b)
- From the beginning the approach taken should be collaborative – that is, the family and other significant others are considered as allies and their expertise is recognized, listened to and valued
- Everyone involved i.e. James, his family members and team members to work collaboratively to identify early warning signs of relapse, review how these may be pre-empted if they occur, develop effective problem solving strategies and examine different methods of communication (Falloon *et al.*, 2004)
- James' mother's concerns and needs to be listened to and acted upon. The team needs to find a way to meet with her, address her personal needs and requests, and work towards involving her more in James' care
- Team members to feedback unmet service needs to their managers and explore the possibilities of restructuring existing services, or to ascertain how existing resources could be reinvested. For example, if some team members could work more flexibly, to include working 'out of office' hours, then they could meet James' mother when she has finished work (and other users and carers with similar needs). Indeed many community mental health teams in the UK do now offer 'out of hour' services, in line with national mental health policy (Department of Health, 2001)
- The organisation should review shortfalls in service provision for family through a needs-mapping exercise and an analysis of other local services. Such an evaluation should be collaborative with local user and carer groups and/or representatives. There is compelling evidence that the involvement of users and carers in mental health research and service evaluation provides more sensitive and accurate information about the impact of treatment(s) and services received (Rose, 2001; Allam *et al.*, 2004). As commented by Repper and Perkins (2003), if services are to use evidence-based practice and thus promote recovery, the

expertise of people who have experienced mental health problems (and their carers) must be the primary force guiding their development.

Conclusion

This case scenario has attempted to address how PSI, with the necessary resources, people and enabling structures in place, can be implemented in practice. However, it needs to be acknowledged that many users and carers will not currently gain access to professionals and teams who have been trained in PSI approaches; their numbers still remain small and are concentrated in localities where PSI training courses have been established (Brooker *et al.*, 2003). Taking the example of specialist early intervention in psychosis (EIP) teams, which are currently being set up to work with young people experiencing their first episode of psychosis, the highly skilled workforce required for these teams is already considered scarce (Sainsbury Centre for Mental Health, 2003). However, training programmes in EIP are currently under development across England and the number of PSI-based courses also continues to rise, although greater national coordination regarding this development is urgently required (Brooker *et al.*, 2003; Sainsbury Centre for Mental Health, 2003).

Another significant implementation problem is that even when there are PSI-trained staff in an organisation, they are not always supported or given the time to practice psychosocial interventions effectively. Taking family intervention as an example, despite the overwhelming research evidence that working with families is highly effective, this psychosocial intervention is not being used to its full potential in clinical practice because: a) there is a lack of trained professionals; and b) for those who are trained, often there is a lack of support within organisations to implement family work (Midence, 2000). A number of follow-up studies of the impact of training programmes (e.g. Kavanagh *et al.*, 1993; Fadden, 1997) have found that organisational and structural barriers have acted as obstacles to the implementation of the approach by professionals. Such barriers have included: failures to provide adequate time for practitioners to carry out family work and receive clinical supervision; difficulties in integrating family work with existing clinical responsibilities, such as high caseloads; availability of time in lieu or overtime for appointments out of hours (as illustrated in the case scenario); and a lack of support from managers.

Finally, we wish to make some comments regarding the future of psychosocial interventions in mental health care. There is no doubt that the research, education and training to date has re-introduced the 'psychosocial' into the way that people with severe mental health problems are cared for today, although it is acknowledged that there are still organisational and structural barriers to the widespread implementation of PSI to be addressed. However, we believe that the PSI approach has provided a philosophy and new way of working with people with severe mental health problems. In doing so, traditional systems and approaches towards people with mental health problems have begun to be challenged. Now a greater emphasis is being placed upon promoting therapeutic hope, intervening earlier and engendering the concept of recovery, resulting in 'a far more rounded, creative approach, which is individually focused and sensitive to the needs of users, particularly young people' (Reeves, 2000: 334). However, whether the PSI approach continues to play a role in mental health care will depend on whether practitioners, their managers, organisations, users and carers continue to embrace the philosophy of PSI and the way of working it promotes – this remains the underlying challenge.

References

Allam, S., Blyth, S., Fraser, A., Hodgson, S., Howes, J., Repper, J. and Newman, A. (2004), 'Our experience of collaborative research: Service users, carers and researchers work together to evaluate an assertive outreach service', *Journal of Psychiatric and Mental Health Nursing*, **11**, 365-373.

Baker, P. (2003), *The Voice Inside: A Practical Guide to Coping with Hearing Voices*. Manchester, Hearing Voices Network (also available on the Mind website: www.mind.org.uk/Information/Booklets/The+voice+inside.htm).

Barrowclough, C. and Tarrier, N. (1992), *Families of Schizophrenic Patients: Cognitive Behavioural Intervention*, London: Chapman and Hall.

Beeforth, M., Conlan, E. and Grayley, R. (1994), *Have We Got Views for You: User Evaluation of Case Management*, London: Sainsbury Centre for Mental Health.

Bentall, R. (2003), *Madness Explained: Psychosis and Human Nature*, Penguin: Allen Lane.

Birchwood, M. (1996), 'Early intervention in psychotic relapse: Cognitive approaches to detection and management', in Haddock, G. and Slade, P.D. (eds), *Cognitive-Behavioural Interventions with Psychotic Disorders*. London: Routledge.

Birchwood, M., Fowler. D. and Jackson, C. (2000), *Early Intervention in Psychosis: A Guide to Concepts, Evidence and Interventions*, Chichester: John Wiley & Sons.

Brooker, C., Falloon, I., Butterworth, C., Goldberg, D., Graham-Hole, V. and Hillier, V. (1994), The outcome of training CPNs to deliver psychosocial interventions, *British Journal of Psychiatry*, 165, 222-230.

Brooker, C., Saul, C., Robinson, J. King, J and Dudley, M. (2003), 'Is training in psychosocial interventions worthwhile? Report of a psychosocial intervention trainee follow-up study', *International Journal of Nursing Studies*, 40, 731-747.

Brown, G.W., Birley, J.L.T. and Wing, J.K. (1972), 'Influence of family life on the Course of Schizophrenic Disorders: A replication', *British Journal of Psychiatry*, 121: 241-63.

Budd, R.J. and Hughes, C.T. (1997), 'What do relatives of people with schizophrenia find helpful about family intervention?', *Schizophrenia Bulletin*, 23(2) 341-347.

Carrick, R., Mitchell, A., Powell, R.A. and Lloyd, K. (2004), 'The quest for well-being: A qualitative study of the experience of taking antipsychotic medication', *Psychology and Psychotherapy: Theory, Research and Practice* 77, 19-33.

Chadwick, P., Trower, P. and Birchwood, M. (1996), *Cognitive Therapy for Delusions, Voices and Paranoia*, Chichester, UK: John Wiley & Sons.

Clinton, M. and Nelson, S. (1996), *Mental Health and Nursing Practice*, Sydney: Prentice Hall.

Day, J.C., Wood, G., Dewey, M. and Bentall, R.P. (1995), 'A self-rating scale for measuring neuroleptic side-effects – validation in a group of schizophrenic patients', *British Journal of Psychiatry*, 166, 650-653.

Department of Health (1990), *The Care Programme Approach for People with a Mental Illness, Referred to Specialist Psychiatric Services. HC (90) 23/LASSA (90) 11*. London: Joint Health and Social Services Circular, Department of Health.

Department of Health (2001), *The Mental Health Policy Implementation Guide*, London: HMSO.

Drury, V. (2000), Cognitive Behaviour Therapy in Early Psychosis in: Birchwood, M., Fowler, D. and Jackson, C. (eds), *Early Intervention in Psychosis: A Guide to Concepts, Evidence and Interventions*, Chichester, UK: John Wiley & Sons, pp. 185-212.

Fadden, G. (1997), 'Implementation of family interventions in routine clinical practice following staff training programmes: A major cause for concern', *Journal of Mental Health*, 6, 599-612.

Falloon, I., Mueser, K., Gingerich, S., Rappaport, S., McGill, C., Graham-Hole,V., Fadden, G. and Gair, F. (2004), *Family Work Manual*, Meriden: The West Midlands Family Programme.

Falloon, I.R.H. and Graham-Hole, V. (1994), *Comprehensive Management of Mental Disorders*, Buckingham: Buckingham Mental Health Service.

Faulkner, A. and Layzell, S. (2000), *Strategies for Living: A Report of User-Led Research into People's Strategies for Living with Mental Distress*, London, Mental Health Foundation.

Fowler, P., Garety, P. and Kuipers, L. (1995), *Cognitive Behavioural Therapy for Psychosis, A Clinical Handbook*, Chichester: John Wiley & Sons.

Fox, J. and Conroy, P. (2000), 'Assessing clients' needs: The semistructured interview', in Gamble, C. and Brennan, G. (eds), *Working with Serious Mental Illness. A Manual for Clinical Practice*, London: Baillière Tindall, pp. 85-96.

Furlong, M. and Leggart. M. (1996), 'Reconciling the patients right to confidentially and the families need to know', *Australian and New Zealand Journal of Psychiatry*, 30, 614-622.

Francell., E.G. (2002), Medication: The foundation of recovery. www.psychlaws.org/generalresources/PA3.HTM.

Gamble, C. (1995), 'The Thorn Nursing Initiative', *Nursing Standard*, 9(15) 31-34.

Gamble, C. (1997), 'The Thorn Nursing Programme: Its past, present and future', *Mental Health Care*, **1**(3) 95-97.

Gamble, C. and Brennan, G. (2000a), 'Assessments: A rationale and glossary of tools', in Gamble, C. and Brennan, G. (eds), *Working with Serious Mental Illness. A Manual for Clinical Practice*, London: Baillière Tindall, pp. 68-84.

Gamble, C. and Brennan, G. (2000b), 'Working with families and informal carers', in Gamble, C. and Brennan, G. (eds), *Working with Serious Mental Illness: A Manual for Clinical Practice*, London: Baillière Tindall, pp. 179-198.

Gray, R., Wykes, T., Parr, A-M., Hails, E. and Gournay, K. (2001), 'The use of outcome measures to evaluate the efficacy and tolerability of antipsychotic medication: A comparison of Thorn graduate and CPN practice', *Journal of Psychiatric and Mental Health Nursing*, 8, 191-196.

Gray, R., Wykes, T. and Gournay, K. (2003), 'The effect of medication management training on community mental health nurse's clinical skills', *International Journal of Nursing Studies*, 40, 163-169.

Intagliata, J. (1982), 'Improving the quality of community care for the chronically mentally disabled: The role of case management', *Schizophrenia Bulletin*, 8: 655-674.

Initiative to Reduce the Impact of Schizophrenia (IRIS), www.iris-initiative.org.uk.

Kanter, J. (1989), 'Clinical case management: Definition, principles, components', *Hospital and Community Psychiatry*, 40: 361-368.

Kavanagh, D.J., Piatokowska, O., Clark, D., O'Halloran, P., Manicavasagar, V., Rosen, A. and Tennant, C. (1993), 'Application of cognitive behavioural family intervention for schizophrenia in multidisciplinary teams: What can the matter be?', *Australian Psychologist*, 23(3), 181-188.

Kuipers, L., Leff, J. and Lam, D. (1992), *Family Work for Schizophrenia: A Practical Guide*, London: Gaskell/Royal College of Psychiatrists.

Lancashire, S., Haddock, G., Tarrier, N., Bagley, I., Butterworth, T. and Brooker, C. (1997), 'Effects of training in psychosocial interventions for community psychiatric nurses in England', *Psychiatric Services*, 48(1) 39-41.

Leach, J. (2003), *Oxford Student Mental Health Network Final Report*, Oxford: Oxford Brookes University, www.brookes.ac.uk/student/services/osmhn/about-osmhn/Reports/Freport.PDF.

Leff, J., Sharpley, M., Chisholm, D., Bell, R. and Gamble, G. (2001), 'Training community psychiatric nurses in schizophrenia family work: A study of clinical and economic outcomes for patients and relatives', *Journal of Mental Health*, 10(2), 189-197.

Leff, J. and Vaughn, C. (1985), *Expressed Emotion in Families*, New York: Guildford.

Lelliott, P., Beevor, A., Hogman, G., Hyslop, J., Lathlean, J. and Ward, M. (2001), 'Carers' and Users' Expectations of Services – User version (CUES-U): A new instrument to measure the experience of users of mental health services', *British Journal of Psychiatry*, 179, 67-72.

Marks, I.M., Connolly, J., Muijen, M., Audini, B., McNamee, G. and Lawrence, R.E. (1994), 'Home-based versus hospital-based care for people with serious mental illness', *British Journal of Psychiatry*, 165, 179-194.

Midence, K. (2000), 'An introduction to and rationale for psychosocial interventions', in Gamble, C. and Brennan, G. (eds), *Working with Serious Mental Illness: A Manual for Clinical Practice*, London: Baillière Tindall, pp. 11-28.

Mills, J. (2000), 'Dealing with voices and strange thoughts', in Gamble, C. and Brennan, G. (eds), *Working with Serious Mental Illness: A Manual for Clinical Practice*, London: Baillière Tindall, pp. 125-162.

MIND (website accessed 27/09/04), User Centred Mental Health Assessments (The Avon Mental Health Measure), www.mind.org.uk/Information/Factsheets/User+empowerment/User+Empowerment+2.htm.

Mueser, K., Bond, G., Drake, R. and Resnick S. (1998), 'Models of community care for severe mental illness: A review of research on case management', *Schizophrenia Bulletin*, 24(1), 37-74.

National Schizophrenia Fellowship, Manic Depression Fellowship and Mind (2001), *That's Just Typical*, NSF, London. www.rethink.org/information/research/That%27s-just-typical.html.

National Schizophrenia Fellowship, Manic Depression Fellowship and Mind (2002), *Doesn't it Make you Sick?* NSF, London. www.rethink.org/information/research/Doesn%27t-it-make-you-sick.htm.

Neuchterlein, K.H., Dawson, M.E. (1984), 'A heuristic vulnerability/stress model of schizophrenic episodes', *Schizophrenia Bulletin*, 10(2), 300-312.

Perry, A., Tarrier, N., Morriss, R., McCarthy, E. and Limb, K. (1999), 'Randomised controlled trial of efficacy of teaching patients with bipolar disorder to identify early symptoms of relapse and obtain treatment', *British Medical Journal*, 318, 149-153.

Pharoah, F.M., Rathbone, J., Mari, J.J. and Streiner, D. (2003), Family intervention for schizophrenia (Cochrane Review), in, *The Cochrane Library*, Issue 4, Chichester, UK: John Wiley & Sons.

Rapp, C. (1998), *The Strengths Model: Case Management with People Suffering from Severe and Persistent Mental Illness*, Oxford, Oxford University Press.

Reeves, A. (2000), Creative Journeys of Recovery: A survivor perspective, in Birchwood, M., Fowler. D. and Jackson, C. (eds), *Early Intervention in Psychosis: A guide to concepts, evidence and interventions*, Chichester: John Wiley & Sons, pp. 327-347.

Repper, D. and Brooker, C. (2002), *Avoiding the Washout: Developing the Organisational Context to Increase the Up Take of Evidence-based Practice for Psychosis*, Northern Centre for Mental health: Durham, www.ncmh.org.uk.

Repper, J., Ford, R. and Cooke, A. (1994), 'How can nurses build trusting relationships with people who have severe and long-term mental health problems? Experiences of case managers and their clients', *Journal of Advanced Nursing*, **19**, 1096-1104.

Repper, J. and Perkins, R. (2003), *Social Inclusion And Recovery: A Model for Mental Health Practice*, London: Baillière Tindall.

Roome, M.A.J. and Escher, A.D. (eds) (1993), *Accepting Voices*, London: Mind Publications.

Roome, M.A.J. and Escher, A.D. (2000), *Making Sense of Voices: A Guide for Mental Health Professionals Working with Voice Hearers*, London: Mind Publications.

Rose, D. (2001), *Users' Voices. The Perspectives of Mental Health Service Users on Community and Hospital Care*, London: Sainsbury Centre for Mental Health.

Sainsbury Centre for Mental Health (2003), *A Window of Opportunity: A Practical Guide for Developing Early Intervention in Psychosis Services*, London: Sainsbury Centre for Mental Health.

Schneider, J., Carpenter, J. and Brandon, T. (1999), 'Operation and organisation of services for people with severe mental illness in the UK: A survey of the Care Programme Approach', *British Journal of Psychiatry*, 175, 422-425.

Simpson, A., Miller, C. and Bowers, L. (2003a), 'Case management models and the care programme approach: How to make the CPA effective and credible', *Journal of Psychiatric and Mental Health Nursing*, 10: 472-483.

Simpson, A., Miller, C. and Bowers, L. (2003b), 'The history of the Care Programme Approach in England: Where did it all go wrong?', *Journal of Mental Health*, 12(5): 489-504.

Sin, J. and Gamble, C. (2003), 'Managing side-effects to the optimum: Valuing a client's experience', *Journal of Psychiatric and Mental Health Nursing*, 10, 147-153.

Social Services Inspectorate (1999), *Still Building Bridges: The Report of a National Inspection of Arrangements for the Integration of Care Programme Approach with Care Management*, London: Department of Health Circular CI (99) 3.

Stein, L.I. and Test, M.A. (1980), 'Alternative to mental hospital treatment 1. Conceptual model, treatment program and clinical evaluation', *Archives of General Psychiatry*, 37, 392-397.

Szmukler, G.I. and Bloch, S. (1997), 'Family involvement in the care of people with psychosis', *British Journal of Psychiatry*, 171, 401-405.

Teschinsky, U. (2000), 'Living with schizophrenia: The family illness experience', *Issues in Mental Health Nursing*, 21, 387-396.

Turner, D. (2001), *Recovery in NSF: 'Wild Geese'*, Internal report for Rethink, www.rethink.org/recovery/Recovery-in-NSF.pdf.

Willets, L.E. and Leff, J. (1997), 'Expressed emotion and schizophrenia: The efficacy of a staff training programme', *Journal of Advanced Nursing*, 26, 1125-1133.

Zubin, J. and Spring, B. (1977), 'Vulnerability: A new view of schizophrenia', *Journal of Abnormal Psychology*, 86, 260-266.

Chapter 15

Spirituality and Mental Health:
An Integrative Dimension

Phil Barker and Poppy Buchanan-Barker

*The person on the spiritual quest for God or enlightenment is like a fish in the sea
looking for the ocean.*

Hide and Seek

We received an invite recently to join a retreat-come-spiritual workshop on some
Greek island. For just under a thousand pounds we could continue the process of
finding the god-within, if not actually become any more certain of the Almighty,
the Ultimate Fountain of Knowledge and Love. It was probably good value for
money but quite why we needed 'this beautiful island' with its numerous 'ancient
sites', and 'spiritual ambience', to discover something about ourselves, escaped us.
Given that the 'self' – whatever that might be – is here and now, 'self-knowledge'
must be waiting, here and now, to be called into our awareness of being. This is the
beginning and end of the problem of this chapter.

If we need to go looking for 'the spiritual' we shall have already missed the
boat or lost the plot – pick your favourite metaphor for pointlessness. We were
probably two of the very few hippies of the 1960s who didn't take an acid 'trip'
through our inner space, or tramp the dusty trail to Kathmandu on the guru trip.
Like today's poor little Nemo, all at sea in the big ocean, or (from our childhood),
Dorothy and Toto chased up the yellow brick road by the Wicked Witch of the
West, we believed that, given sufficient attendance at the School of Hard Knocks,
we all might realise that 'home is best'– more of which later. And anyway, we
were too busy just doing and being. Living can offer a great education, especially
when you are young and broke.

Like Gertrude Stein we intuited that wherever we were headed, when we got
there, there would probably be no 'there', *there*. One doesn't have to be a Zen
Buddhist to get this joke, but it helps. Discovering the infinite, effing the ineffable
or just finding one's place in the cosmos, is as much about *making sense* of things,
as any other form of education (*educere*: to draw out from within). We simply
come to know better what we already know. Wisdom is a visitor not a destination.

Whether we view ourselves as shaped by the Hand of God or a complex
molecular orchestration chaotically evolved within the universe, our deepest

understandings come from within. When Stephen Hawking talked about 'knowing the mind of god' he might have been playing with scientific metaphor, but he was also repeating the aspirations of many a theologian or mystic. *Knowing* is felt in our total being. Invariably it is near impossible to represent this experience in words. Genuine learning shares the same space. Everything else, as Einstein quipped, is mere information.

The reader may struggle with this chapter and may even raise a little spiritual sweat. Certainly our intention is not to inform. Modern psychiatry and psychology is replete with people claiming to 'know'; hell-bent on force-feeding others with their personal take on being and becoming human. We offer only our take of other people's stories. The simple *truth* – as opposed to fact – of spirituality is that people already have all that they need to embark on and explore the spiritual dimension. Everything else – this chapter included – is commerce. No guru – no method – no teacher.

Daydream Believers

Spirituality is rapidly gaining credence in the world of mental health, as more and more people who struggle to make sense of their experience of madness, turn to the language of the 'spiritual' to express something of the complexity of the alienating states, so laughably called 'mental health problems'. People may not know what has upset their lives, knocked them for six, or otherwise is *ailing* them, but attributing it to the disturbing effects of biochemistry (biological), dysfunctional belief systems (psychological), childhood upbringing (social) or all three (biopsychosocial), is not far removed from the old practice of attributing madness to possession by demons. The contemporary scientific 'explanations' allegedly reduce stigma, by showing that the person is not responsible. However, people didn't actually invite the 'demons' either, so where does that leave us?

If one removes the new language, not much has changed in the madness business. In our youth, in the 1950s, there were just over 100 forms of madness. Today there are close on 400. So, in a categorical sense, we are four times as crazy (Kirk and Kutchins, 1997). Apart from sidestepping the lunacy of diagnosis, spirituality may also be attractive for its timelessness, finding echoes in poetry, literature, opera and the visual arts; if not also magic, ritual and humankind's primeval relationship to time and place. When spoken aloud in public, or expressed in print, spirituality triggers some powerful resistance, especially for its assumed relationship with organised religion.

It is rarely the believers who get upset by loose talk of spirituality, although some 'faiths' have become so secular that any suggestions that people might experience the divine, is viewed as sacrilege. It is usually lapsed Christians, or those trying to escape the domestic tagging of Judaism, who become overheated: protesting the meaningless babble of spirituality, its associations with everything 'New Age', or simply that they 'don't understand it!' This final protest is – ironically – the whole point.

Spirituality – especially in the 'mental health' context – is all about journey and unceasing exploration. It is a long way from anything as simple as *understanding*. The 'spiritual' is the antithesis of the Mary Poppins of Rationality. Instead of offering the reassurance of logic, spirituality impersonates Scrooge's ghostly Christmas visitors: beckoning us to look beyond the veneer of our lives; rummaging through the tidily ordered constructs that frame our existence. Nothing necessarily is what it seems, although it *might* be so, spiritual discourse seems to say. We might well be dreaming we are butterflies, or we might be butterflies dreaming we are human. Who knows? Whoever does isn't telling.

Brainless or Mindless?

Spirituality is also an intellectual problem. Shrouded in enigma, it refuses to be classified, categorised or measured. This upsets the empirically minded who, like Francis Crick, think that *who* we are – in this neuroscientifically fascinated age – involves no more than brain function. Crick famously observed that:

> You, your joys and sorrows, your memories and ambitions, your sense of personal identity and free will, are in fact no more than the behaviour of a vast assembly of nerve cells and their associated molecules (Crick, 1995: 3).

Crick believed that this was a new idea but, as Szasz (1996) noted, this was just because he was ignorant of the history of the mind and especially of madness. Notably, Crick insisted that his approach to the problem of the mind was scientific but this was:

> a claim he supports by denying agency to persons and attributing agency to things. In Crick's world, neural networks 'learn' and Free Will (capitalized) is an attribute of the cerebral cortex. He asks: 'Where might Free Will be located in the brain?' and answers: 'Free Will is located in or near the anterior cingulated sulcus' (Szasz, 1996: 84).

Crick's search for the root of human stories, is akin to taking the television apart, expecting to find the actors (and the script) from some soap-opera *in* its processors and circuitry. They must be in *here* somewhere? Where else could they be?

Crick, along with James Watson, unraveled the mysteries of DNA. So, in one sense he ought to know 'who' we are – being one of the cleverest minds at the cutting edge of consciousness research. Crick is one of neuroscience's bully-boys, intent on bashing a very big hole in the traditional Western idea of the 'self'. However, Crick confuses 'what' people are with 'who' they, and others, believed them to be. In that space of being lies our identity as *persons*. The mind is like a rippling pool. The ripples clearly belong to the property called water but are clearly not caused by water itself. The idea that might trace the ultimate location of some of the rippling characteristics of who and what we are, as persons – to the anterior cingulated sulcus – simply doesn't hold water.

We are stories. As long as we live people will tell stories about us, and we will tell stories about our-selves. Who we *are*, at least as social animals, lies in a grey space somewhere between those stories. As Frankl (2000) carefully argued, we are biological, psychological and social stories – but we are also more than that. As humans we write, edit, tell and retell our story of what it *means* to have these different bodily, mental and social experiences. Stones, trees and animals may also have meaningful stories about their existence but as yet we have found no way of accessing them. Humans, on the other hand, have been telling stories about life and its meaning (however rich or banal) since we were able to engage in meaningful discourse. Our ancestors' attempts to re-present the world outside their bodies, in cave paintings and crude carvings, were one good example. Whether or not they 'knew' the significance of what they were doing is unimportant. That they did so is significance itself.

When 'mad' people talk, write poems, or otherwise try to represent, however crudely or artistically, their experience of madness, they engage in similar meaning-making. Of course the context has changed greatly. Even as we write this chapter, we cannot claim that these words belong to us – at least not entirely. Our stories are connected invisibly to so many others stories about us, told by others; and other people's stories about themselves, which have influenced us down the years. And we haven't even begun to consider the stories about Phil and Poppy as men or women, sons and daughters, Scots, as descendants of the Celtic peoples, working class émigrés – the list is potentially endless. However, all these stories *about* us, pale into insignificance, when we confront the fundamentals of *who* and *what* we are, as *persons*.

The stories that are told, revised, updated, and edited, *about* mentally ill or otherwise *mad* people shares the same territory. These stories – from the 'grand narratives' of psychiatric diagnosis to the often highly subjective accounts written in case notes, court reports or other clinical files – may well be *about* the person, but – even when honest and well-intentioned – are not *of* the person. These stories lie beyond the domain of personhood – where those people (as opposed to the patients/clients/users or consumers they are presumed to be) actually live out their lives.

More and more people caught in the myriad nets of madness have come to repeat Frankl's epiphany: realising that ultimately they must define themselves. This act of self-definition ultimately belongs to the world of the spirit, where all cultures, however sophisticated or primitive, assume that the soul or psyche resides. It is strangely ironic that the shiny sane minds of our day – like Francis Crick – can see no further than the molecular goo of our organic selves. Were he to look a bit further – diving through the molecular gate to the sub-atomic level – he would find that, ultimately there is nothing there but the void: the great emptiness. And, like many who have voyaged through madness, sinking through the depths to experience their own 'nothingness', Crick might realise that the void that lies beneath, is the same Void that lies beyond our human experience of Self. The great enigma – that everything exists in nothing – might not reveal anything new but certainly puts a new slant on the notion that *all* we *are* is pulsing grey matter.

All Alone: Fear, Losing and Loathing

Psychic suffering takes many forms. Threaded through much human distress is the ancient and pervasive spectre of *fear*. Meditating on the grief he felt after his wife's death C.S. Lewis (1961) observed:

> *No one ever told me that grief felt so like fear. I am not afraid, but the sensation is like being afraid. The same fluttering in the stomach, the same restlessness, the yawning. I keep on swallowing (Lewis, 1961: 61).*

The experience of loss reminds us that the final threat we face is our ultimate *aloneness*. In *The Rime of the Ancient Mariner*, Coleridge offered a metaphor for humankind's blind rejection of everything that lies beyond our existing knowledge. Anything, not already part of our received wisdom, is to be feared and, if possible, controlled. By killing the albatross, the *youthful* mariner was forced to face the emptiness of his isolate existence:

> *Alone, alone, all, all alone,*
> *Alone on a wide, wide sea!*
> *And never a saint took pity on*
> *My soul in agony.*

Only with time, and the wisdom of hindsight did the, by now *ancient*, mariner come to understand the meaning of his once bloody act. Coleridge's poetry and philosophical writing was shot through with self-doubt and a metaphysical anxiety that anticipated modern existentialism. Although hardly a spiritual text, Coleridge's poem carries some important messages about experience, fear, responsibility and humankind's almost insignificant scale on the wider canvas of existence. People may not be responsible for their madness – although some might well be – but they are responsible for their experience of it. That responsibility can become, for some, like an albatross, especially in these responsibility-shirking times.

The success story of contemporary mental health is the continued rise of mutual support groups, survivor groups and especially Survivor Poetry groups. Through sharing their experiences of madness, these people appear to remedy their sense of aloneness. Through personal reflection they appear to come to know it better *and* differently. Most people who encounter madness look for some explanation: what is happening to me? Where did this come from? What does this mean? Typically the person is offered a diagnosis, intended to explain *and* diminish the distress. But, what is such re-assurance really worth? As Szasz once famously quipped: 'I thought I was going crazy but then I found out it was just schizophrenia'. The truth of the matter must involve more than simply re-labelling. Maybe writing a stanza or two is worth more than genuflecting before the DSM IV.

Psychiatry and the Soul

Originally, psychiatry sought to study the soul, although many of those who cast themselves as 'psychiatric survivors' might be forgiven for laughing aloud at this historical relic (Newnes, Holmes and Dunn, 2000). The soul has fallen through the floor of mainstream psychiatry, although a tiny number of psychiatrists are trying to reinstate this ancient focus (Culliford, 2002). If we wanted to be pedantic we would simply ask – how could psychiatry exist without examining the spiritual. However, the turbulence of the past 100 years has muddied the psychiatric waters and the spiritual focus is, at least for the moment, obscured from view.

The psychotherapeutic arm of psychiatry followed, perhaps unwittingly, the path recommended by the Buddha and Socrates who both suggested the power of 'looking within': examining life as a way of revealing meaning. Indeed, understanding life and our part *of* it, and *in* it, may be both the beginning and end of the spiritual journey that *begins* in psychotherapy, but cannot be completed in such an ultimately *mundane* activity.

The person caught in the spiral of madness tries, desperately, to return to wholeness – feeling as if they are threatened with complete disintegration. For many, this begins with self-realisation and the search for meaning, exploring, as LeShan (1999) observed, the states of being that appear to use the most of themselves. Traditional psychiatry and psychotherapy uses, instead, a historical-pathological approach, trying to establish how the person 'became' like this. Instead, we should be exploring what this whole process of collapse and disintegration might be about, its hidden meanings, and what the person might be trying to *accomplish* within the spiritual crisis.

By emphasising his belief that what *really matters* is not the particular school of psychotherapy, but the openness, humility and even ignorance, of the therapist, Karasu (2001) challenged the traditional professional empire of psychotherapy and psychiatry. In his most recent work, Karasu (2003) has acknowledged that material possessions, success, power and pleasure often fail to fill the void that lies at the heart of our lives. For many, the life of a 'spiritual tourist' (Brown, 1998) offers some reassurance but, ultimately, the hollow feeling that 'something is missing' returns. As far as Karasu is concerned, we have no option but to begin to explore the deepest yearnings of our heart. Especially in the West, our greatest yearning may be for 'happiness' (Whiteside, 2001) but, as Karasu noted, there is no end to the journey to 'real happiness'. Indeed, there is not even a good place to start. Karasu urges us to start *here*, where we are, to begin the journey NOW!

This echoes the traditional Eastern (especially Buddhist) emphasis on *embracing* rather than denying, the painful aspects of our lives. The fear of loss – especially of our 'sanity' and selfhood – may lie at the very heart of the spiritual vacuum of our lives, and may even deter us from taking that first, necessary, step into the next moment.

Mental Health and Meaning

But what has any of this do with 'mental health'? In the USA the Surgeon General (1999) defined mental health as:

> ... the successful performance of mental function, resulting in productive activities, fulfilling relationships with other people, and the ability to adapt to change and cope with adversity (US Dept Health, 1999: 171).

Note the emphasis on *function* and *efficacy*. By implication, anyone not *productively* engaged, or who experiences *unfulfilling* relationships or who experiences even the occasional flutter of disquiet in the face of everyday challenges, *cannot* be mentally healthy. As with all such bureaucratic definitions of health and well-being, one is left wondering who does fit these stringent criteria?

The past decade has witnessed a switch of emphasis from the concept of 'mental health' to the facilitation of recovery (Anthony, 1993). The emphasis on growing through and beyond the experience of distress and especially the focus on *meaning* seems to redefine the mental health agenda, bringing it closer to a consideration of the 'point' of a person's life. Such a *point* might involve not only questing for meaning in life, but also – as Frankl (2000) argued – begging whether any such meanings exist at all. Such an emphasis on shifts our focus beyond the internal functioning alluded to in most bureaucratic definitions of mental health, to an appreciation of the almost ineffable, emergent story of the person's life (Leibrich, 1999).

For Leibrich, meaning is always *there* – in the story of our lives – whether we are aware of it or not. The journey of recovery may be no more than the long walk to recognition of that meaning. For us, the journey is often taken on uncharted seas, invoking the dangers of the deep as well as of distance. Leibrich (1999) sees the story as a gift, even when it involves the pain of madness.

> The act of telling stories can restore people ('re-store'). The telling of our story to someone who is genuinely interested and who relates to the telling through their own experiences is a very precious thing (Leibrich, 1999: 5).

The story makes its own journey in search of greater understanding, which may be found in the genuine listener. This explains in some way why people 'talk to God' and often claim to have been 'heard' (O'Brien, 1964).

This sense of communication is echoed in most commonly accepted definitions of spirituality, which is often understood to involve some kind of a partnership with one's Higher Power or Godhead or Nature. As Culliford (2002) noted, spirituality can provide hope and solace during the person's crisis or experience of illness. Individually this might take the form of a sense of peace or in groups, a sense of understanding and social support.

Although often projected as being 'un-worldly', the engagement with the spiritual life is a highly practical and grounded activity: in human terms, an essential rather than a luxury. People come to realise that they have no choice *but* to be on the spiritual path, since ultimately the materialist's outlook on life invites us to believe in 'nothing'.

The Celtic Perspective

For us, spirituality is a question without an answer. Something we look for but do not actually expect to find. As we try to live our lives in pursuit of a higher understanding of ourselves, and our place in the universe, we examine all that we know of what is inside and outside of ourselves. In our Celtic spiritual tradition, the journey we take *towards* understanding always leads home. The Celtic Knot symbolises the journey – snaking outwards it eventually loops back to where it started – the hearth of home. John O'Donohue (1997) reminded us that, although we are often told that the spiritual journey involves a sequence of stages, this is an illusion:

> You do not need to go away outside your self to come into real conversation with your soul and the mysteries of your spiritual world. *The eternal is at home* – within you (O'Donohue, 1997: 120, emphasis added).

At the other side of the world, in New Zealand, Julie Leibrich (2001), in a lecture on spirituality found a similar understanding, 'It is a kind of coming home. For me, the meaning of spirituality is meaning itself'. Leibrich's experience may well be signalling an important 'change of heart' in the whole field of spirituality and mental health:

> My definition of mental health has a lot in common with the way I define spirituality. Both concepts are concerned with the experience of self. One reaching into dimensions of space to discover self, the other realising the freedom that comes from accepting self. That is why spiritual experiences and their interpretation can have such a profound influence on mental health (Leibrich, 2001, lecture notes).

Leibrich appreciated that there might be something 'in' the space of her Self that might ultimately be of great value.

No Guru, No Method, No Teacher

So, how do we respond to extreme forms of human distress? When we consider what human distress might 'mean' – in spiritual terms – the wisdom of 'fixing', as opposed to developing understanding, might be questioned. Indeed, many people make discoveries *within* psychotherapy, which appear to have little to do with the therapeutic method, or even the therapist, but may be a function of their own reflection: no more and no less (Barker and Kerr, 2000; Karasu, 2001). In that sense, the therapist – and the therapeutic method – may only be providing a *context*, or setting, for the person to engage in a necessary act of reflecting.

In this consumerist age many therapists now sell their wares on television, marketing themselves and their 'new' methods as the answer to all manner of human ills. The idea that these therapies (and their sophisticated therapists) are unnecessary is a threatening concept. If the Emperor really has no 'new clothes' then people must confront their own individuality, make their own choices, if not their own 'clothes'; as they reflect on their own experience, coming to their own realisation of who they are and what is the ultimate meaning of their lives (Frankl, 2000).

Wrestling with the Angel, on Very Thin Ice

The contemporary pairing of spirituality and mental health may, in years to come, provokes much head scratching. Certainly, the contemporary critic of such a development might well argue that many (if not most) people in states of high anxiety, deep despair or extreme alienation – whether from self or others – are *disturbed*, and that this disturbance lies somewhere, or perhaps in several places, within the physical body. In that sense, not much has changed since Hippocrates' day. However, it could also be said that any 'disturbing' experience shields the potential for spiritual revelation.

What is the difference between the tortured soul of Coleridge's *Ancient Mariner* and the tortured experiences of those who have encountered what has been called madness and now, patronisingly, is referred to as *mental health problems*? Probably not a lot, not as far as we are concerned. However, we would urge caution against simply accepting, at face value, every unusual experience as evidence of an encounter with the Absolute, however we might wish to define this.

Not all 'madness' is a 'spiritual emergence' and vice versa. When the late New Zealand writer, Janet Frame, was given a diagnosis of schizophrenia, and this led to years of futile and damaging psychiatric treatment. The writer, who had experienced a huge number of emotional and spiritual upheavals in her early life, was 'wrestling with the angel' (King, 2001), caught in the eye of the storm of spiritual emergence. She was not crazy.

> Sally Clay (1999) was, by her own admission, *possessed* by madness, yet she too was like Jacob, wrestling with the angel. And so she wrote: 'Jacob named the place of his struggle Peniel, which means "face of God". I too have seen God face to face, and I want to remember my Peniel. I really do not want to be called recovered. From the experience of madness I received a wound that changed my life. It enabled me to help others and to know myself. I am proud that I have struggled with God and with the mental health system. I have not recovered. I have overcome' (King, 2001: 15).

This is the strange, ironic, paradox of madness. The spiritually emergent can *appear* mad, and the completely and utterly crazy can also be staging their own Titanic battle with their demons, if not also their conception of the Absolute Other – whether actual or metaphorical. Who would claim to tell the difference?

Perhaps because we have been fortunate to know, *personally*, people like Sally Clay, we find it easy to accept the *truth* of their apocalyptic struggle. The more we listen, carefully, to tales from the dark side of madness – and also the dark side of mental health 'treatment' – the more the spiritual construction of their plight makes sense. It rings bells in the echoing caverns of our souls. Perhaps these metaphorical 'bells' are not just an interesting musical 'treatment' of the human condition. Perhaps they are part of the human 'wake up call' that is long overdue in so-called mental health *care*.

For most people, the experience of madness is a psychic injury, from which it is often near-impossible to recover. For many, the experience of mental health services is little more than *insult added to injury*. We are now more than 100 years into the 'scientific' era of 'modern psychiatry'. In many senses we are *informed* beyond our wildest imaginings, yet still lacking in even the simplest understanding of what madness might *mean* for the people so afflicted, demonised and tormented.

The concept of spirituality does not offer any 'quick fix' for the meaninglessness of contemporary practice, but it does serve as signpost, pointing us back to the person – the overflowing reservoir of knowledge and potential understanding of whatever is going on under the storm clouds of madness. All we need do is go ask. But first we must gird our own 'spiritual' loins in preparation for what the person's story might mean for us. For the simple truth is that we are not *alone* – only disconnected.

References

Anthony, W.A. (1993), 'Recovery from mental illness: The guiding vision of the mental health service system in the 1990s', *Innovations and Research*, **2**, 17-24.

Barker, P. and Kerr, B. (2000), *The Process of Psychotherapy: The Journey of Discovery*, Oxford: Butterworth Heinemann.

Brown, M. (1998), *The Spiritual Tourist: A Personal Odyssey Through the Outer Reaches of Belief*, Bloomsbury: London.

Clay, S. (1999), 'Madness and reality', in Barker, P., Campbell, P. and Davidson, B. (eds) *From the Ashes of Experience: Reflections on Madness, Recovery and Growth*, Whurr: London.

Crick, F. (1995), *The Astonishing Hypothesis*, New York: Simon and Schuster.

Culliford, L. (2002), 'Spiritual care and psychiatric treatment: An introduction', *Advances in Psychiatric Treatment*, **8**, 249-261.

Frankl, V.E. (2000), *Man's search for Ultimate Meaning*, Cambridge Mass: Perseus Publishing.

Karasu, T.B. (2001), *The Psychotherapist as Healer*, New York: Jason Aaronson.

Karasu, T.B. (2003), *The Art of Serenity*, New York: Simon and Schuster.

King, M. (2001), *Wrestling with the Angel: A Life of Janet Frame*, Picador/Macmillan: London.

Kirk, S.A. and Kutchins, H. (1997), *Making us Crazy: The Psychiatric Bible and the Creation of Mental Disorders*, New York: Free Press.

Leibrich, J. (1999), *A Gift of Stories: Discovering How to Deal with Mental Illness*, University of Otago Press/Mental Health Commission: Dunedin, New Zealand.

Leibrich, J. *Making Space – Spirituality and Mental Health*, The Mary Hemingway Rees Memorial Lecture, World Assembly for Mental Health, Vancouver, July 2001.

LeShan, L. (1999), *Cancer as a Turning Point*, New York: Plume.

Lewis, C.S. (1961), *A Grief Observed*, London: Fontana.

Newnes, C., Homes, G. and Dunn, C. (2000), *This is madness: A Critical Look at Psychiatry and the Future of Mental Health Services*, PCCS Books: Ross-on-Wye, UK.

O'Brien, J.A. (1964), *Eternal Answers for an Anxious Age*, London: WH Allen.

O'Donhue, J. (1997), *Anam Cara: Spiritual Wisdom from the Celtic World*, Bantam Books: London.

Szasz, T.S. (1996), *The Meaning of Mind: Language, Morality and Neuroscience*, London: Praeger.

U.S. Department of Health and Human Services (1999), *Mental Health: A Report of the Surgeon General – Executive Summary*, Rockville, MD: U.S. Department of Health and Human Services, Substance Abuse and Mental Health Services Administration, Center for Mental Health Services, National Institutes of Health, National Institute of Mental Health.

Whiteside, P. (2001), *Happiness: The 30-day Guide*, London: Rider Books.

Index